Textbook of
FORENSIC ODONTOLOGY

Textbook of FORENSIC ODONTOLOGY

KMK Masthan MDS
Professor and Head
Department of Oral Pathology and
Vice Principal (Academics)
Sree Balaji Dental College and Hospital, Chennai
Tamil Nadu, India

JAYPEE

JAYPEE BROTHERS MEDICAL PUBLISHERS
The Health Sciences Publisher
New Delhi | London

Jaypee Brothers Medical Publishers (P) Ltd

Headquarters
EMCA House
23/23-B, Ansari Road, Daryaganj
New Delhi 110 002, India
Landline: +91-11-23272143, +91-11-23272703
+91-11-23282021, +91-11-23245672
E-mail: jaypee@jaypeebrothers.com

Corporate Office
4838/24, Ansari Road, Daryaganj
New Delhi 110 002, India
Phone: +91-11-43574357
Fax: +91-11-43574314
E-mail: jaypee@jaypeebrothers.com

Overseas Office
J.P. Medical Ltd
83 Victoria Street, London
SW1H 0HW (UK)
Phone: +44 20 3170 8910
E-mail: info@jpmedpub.com

EU GPSR Authorised Representative
Logos Europe, 9 rue Nicolas Poussin
17000, La Rochelle, France
Phone: +33 (0) 6 67 93 73 78
E-mail: contact@logoseurope.eu

Website: www.jaypeebrothers.com
Website: www.jaypeedigital.com

Inquiries for bulk sales may be solicited at: jaypee@jaypeebrothers.com

Textbook of Forensic Odontology

First Edition : 2009

Reprint: 2026

ISBN 978-81-8448-683-4

Printed in India

Dedicated to
my daughter Roshan

Foreword

भारतीय दन्त परिषद
DENTAL COUNCIL OF INDIA
(CONSTITUTED UNDER THE DENTISTS ACT 1948)
Aiwan-E-Ghalib Marg, Kotla Road, New Delhi-110 002

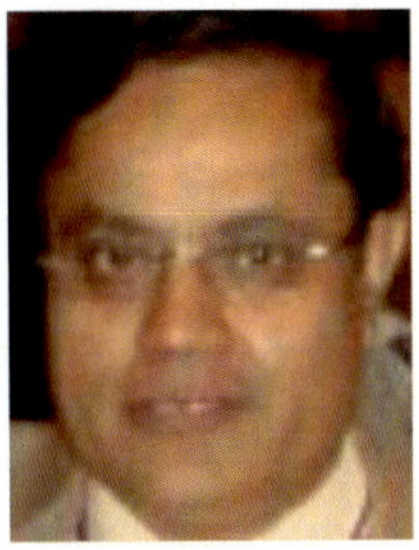

DR. ANIL KOHLI
MDS (Lko), DNBE (USA)
President
Awardee:
- **Padmashri**
- **Padmabhushan**
- **Dr. B.C. Roy National Award**

Telephone : 23220204 (Direct)
: 23238542, 23236740
Fax : 0091 - 11 - 23231252
: 0091 - 11 - 23220204
E-mail : dciindia@hotmail.com
Website : http://www.dciindia.org

No. DE-118-2008/A1626

This *textbook of Forensic Odontology* written by Dr KMK Masthan and his faculty members of Sree Balaji Dental College and Hospital, Chennai is the need to the hour since this subject has been introduced in the 5th year of new BDS curriculum. Forensic Odontology is not elaborately discussed in the existing textbooks of Oral Pathology.

The authors have done extensive spade work and have come out with a simple and easy-to-understand text form of this new discipline for the undergraduate students. The authors have been thorough, dedicated and detailed in the their academic expression.

I wish them all the best for this pioneer task and hope this book becomes the benchmark for other books in this discipline.

(Brig (Dr) Anil Kohli)
MDS (Lko), DNB (USA)
President, Dental Council of India

Preface

Forensic odontology is a new discipline of forensic medicine from a dentist's view point. This has been introduced as a subject for 5th year of new BDS curriculum. A welcome move since this precise and voluminous subject can no longer be studied as a peripheral chapter in oral pathology.

The increasing importance of newer knowledge in forensic odontology is not adequately discussed in the existing textbooks of oral pathology and forensic medicine.

This book is the byproduct of one and half year spade work by the faculty of Department of Oral Pathology, Sree Balaji Dental College, Chennai, Tamil Nadu. I am especially grateful to Dr Shankargouda Patil and Dr Jagadish Prasad Rajguru my postgraduate students for their sincere efforts in bringing out this book.

Through this book,only the tested and commonly accepted theories and hypotheses have been presented. We acknowledge that though this is sufficient for undergraduate students, may not be adequate for postgraduate students.

Lapses and ambiguities may have crept in, which we hope to correct in the further editions of this book. Your suggestions and feedback are welcome at *masthankmk@yahoo.com*

KMK Masthan
M Sathish Kumar
N Aravindha Babu
KT Shanmugam

Contents

CHAPTER 1

Introduction to Forensic Science

DEFINITION

- The word forensic is derived from the Latin word, forensic meaning public. The word science can be defined as systematized knowledge through study using the scientific method. The scientific method is the principles and procedures for the systematic pursuit of knowledge involving the recognition and formulation of a problem, the collection of data through observation and experimentation, and the formulation and testing of hypotheses. Forensic science refers to areas of endeavour that can be used in a judical setting and accepted by the court and the general scientific community to separate truth from untruth.

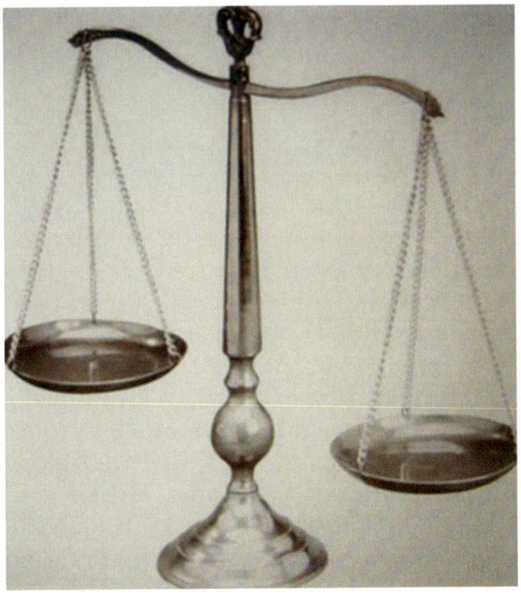

Fig. 1.1

- Forensic odontology can be defined as a branch of dentistry which deals with the proper handling and examination of dental evidence and with the proper evaluation and presentation of dental findings in the interest of dentist.
- Some authors prefer to use the term forensic odontostomatology as its purview includes the whole of orofacial region. The term forensic dentistry is also used interchangeably with forensic odontology.

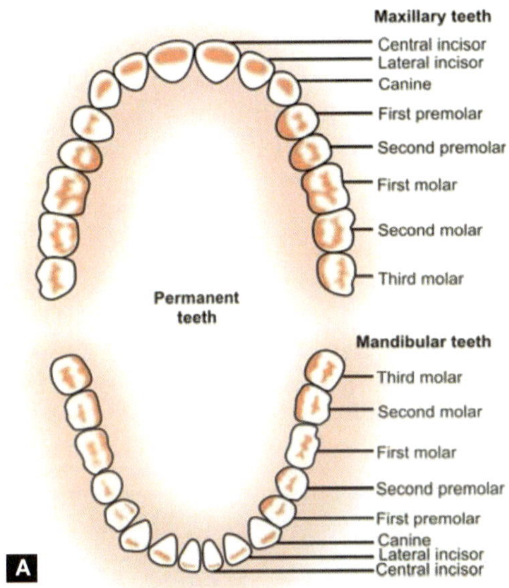

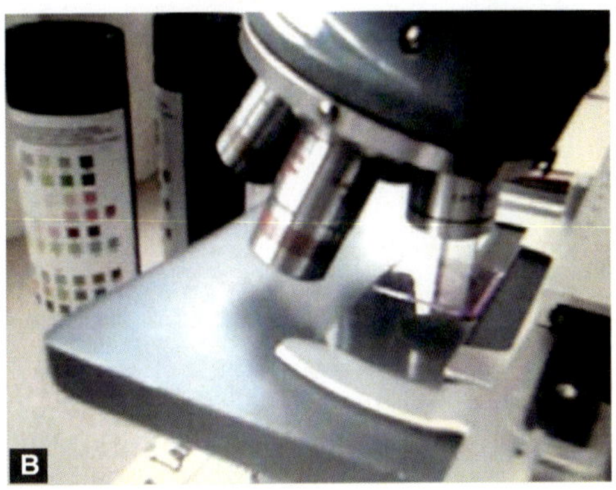

Figs 1.2A and B

HISTORY OF FORENSIC ODONTOLOGY

- Some of the major landmarks in the evolution of forensic dentistry are elaborated here.

- The dentition was, thought to be, used for the first time in 49 AD, in identification of an individual by Agrippina, the wife of Claudius-Roman emperor. She used the peculiar features present in the teeth of her rival and divorcee of her husband, Lollia Poulina, for identification of the body after getting her beheaded.
- Around third century BC the great Indian sage Vatsayana depicted, in detail, the human bitemarks and its classification of skin pertaining to love making for the first time in Indian literature.
- In India, the Rathore raja of Kannauj, Jai Chandra was recognized by his false teeth after he was beaten and killed in the battle. This was, in 1199 AD, probably the first case of identification from dention reported in India. This is given in Elphinstone's "History of India" 5th edition.
- John Talbot, Earl of Shrewsbury, a veteran warrior in his 80's who fell in the battle of Castillion was identified by his teeth in 1453. Dentition also helped to identify the body of Charles the Bold, in 1477, who was found without armor and clothes. The earliest case of bitemark analysis was the Salem trial of 1692, culminated in the conviction of Rev George Boroughs.
- In 1770's Paul Revere, a practicing dentist in US, identified the remains of his friend Dr Joseph Warren from the silver wire fixed bridge made by him. This is thought to be the **first case of identification of a person by a dentist**. The family dentist made a definite identification of John Wilkes Booth's body from dentition to bury the controversies surrounding his death.

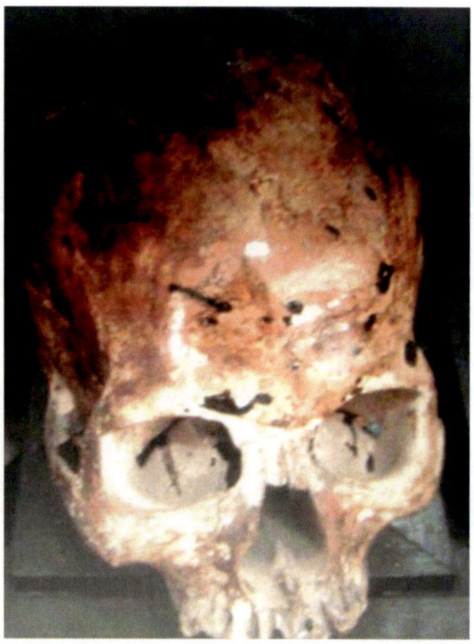

Fig. 1.3

- **Dr Oscar Amoedo,** Professor at a Dental School in Paris, presented a paper entitled "The role of the dentists in the identification of the victims of the catastrophe of the Bazaar de la Charite, Paris, 4 May 1897" at the International Medical Congress of Moscow, he included many of the concepts of dental identification used in the above disaster in his blood "L' Art Dentaire enmedicine Lagale" published in 1898. It was he who suggested the need for an Internationals System of Uniform Charting and a Mutual Understanding of Nomenclature. He is considered as **father of forensic odontology**.
- Advertisements, especially in professional journals, were found to be helpful in assisting the coroner in identifying the victim. It was first used in 1939 by Commissioner Edward J Hickey, who advertised in Journal of American Dental Association. It was seen by a Massachusetts dentist who recognized the bridge constructed by him leading to the identification of the victim and charting the events leading to his death. Later such advertisements appeared in several dental journals like British Dental Journal.
- Dentition was an important lead in the identification of the remains of various leaders who were killed like Zia Ul Haq, former Pakistani president and Rajiv Gandhi, Former Indian Prime Minister. In 1966 Gustafson wrote a comprehensive textbook "Forensic Odontology" which was considered as the Bible in its time. The first format instruction program in forensic dentistry was started at the Armed Forces Institute of Pathology in US in the sixties.

SIGNIFICANCE OF FORENSIC ODONTOLOGY

- Although teeth had been used in the identification of individuals throughout history, mostly as isolated cases, it was never an organized field as it is now. It is perhaps more significant in the present day world. Nowadays a lot of people are found to be missing, dead, murdered or killed in accidents. The identification of these corpses, many a times mutilated bodies, is of paramount importance from a social, emotional and legal view points. Forensic odontology also monitors its own parent profession against malpractice.
- The American Academy of Forensic Sciences, the largest forensic group in the world with a membership of more than 5300 forensic scientists, recognizes 10 areas of forensic endeavor: Criminalistics, engineering science, general, jurisprudence, odontology, pathology/biology, psychiatry and behavior science, questioned documents, toxicology, and physical

anthropology. The pathologist is helpful in determining the time of death by looking at factors such as rigor mortis, livor mortis, postmortem body temperature, decomposition, and chemical changes occuring after death. An autopsy consists of several parts, charting all the external injuries, anatomic dissection, histologic studies, toxicology, and cultures.

FORENSIC DISCIPLINES

- **Criminalistics** is the branch of forensic science involved in the area of laboratory testing of various types of physical evidence, including biologic fluids, DNA, and suspicious chemicals. Criminalists can determine the qualitative and quantitative values of unknown chemicals.

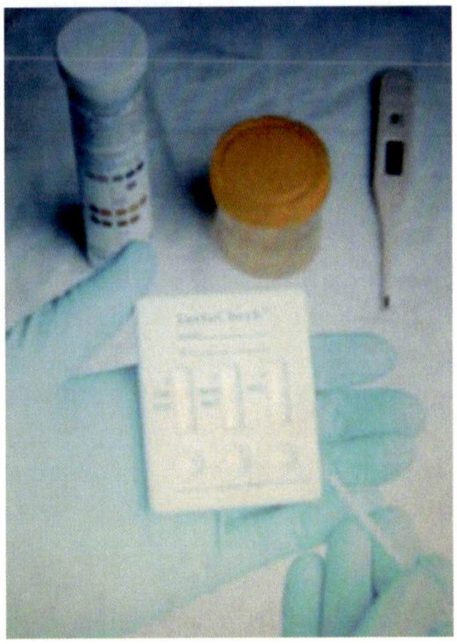

Fig. 1.4

- The field of **engineering science** generally is involved with the structural aspects of a crime scene or accident scene.
- **Jurisprudence** is the area of forensic science dealing with the judicial process and the weight placed on various types of forensic information in adjudicating a legal issue.

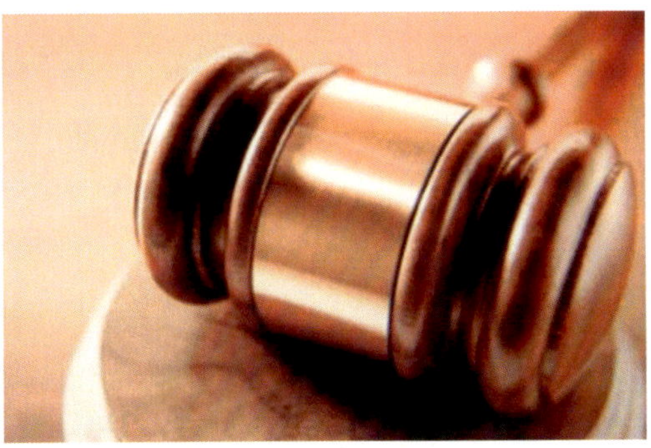

Fig. 1.5

- **Psychiatry and behavior science** is an area of forensic science that studies the behavioral pattern of criminals and often helps the court determine whether a suspect is able mentally to stand trial.
- **Questioned documents** is the area of forensic working with the verification that a written document is what it is purported to be and the signature on the document is authentic.
- **Toxicology** is the field of study involving the testing of drug levels in biologic fluids and their reactions in the human body.

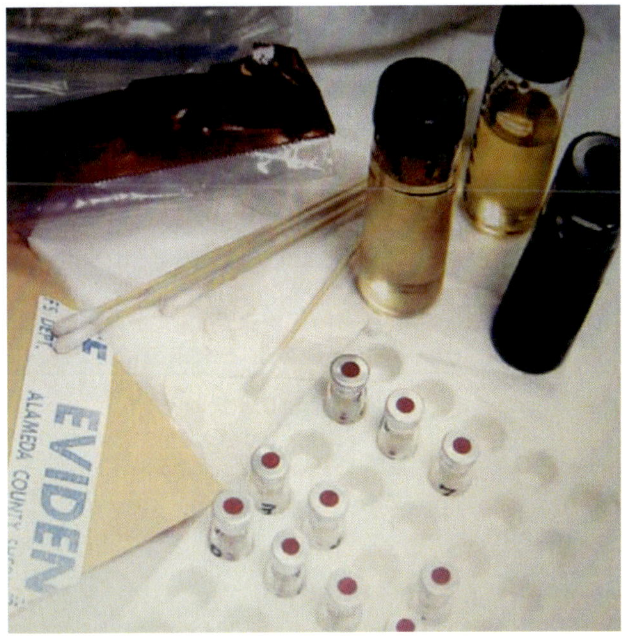

Fig. 1.6

- The **general section** of forensic science includes members that do not fit into the other recognized areas but are involved in the forensic sciences.
- The **physical anthropology** of forensic science deals with the reconstruction of an individual from the bones or skeleton. With their ability to determine the location of grave or burial sites, anthropologists are particularly helpful when a body is buried.
- The **pathology/biology section deals** with the pathologic and physiologic changes of a body before and after death.
- **The autopsy** is a crucial part of many death investigations, helping to determine the cause and manner of death. The cause of death is any injury, disease, metabolic condition, or malformation that plays a part in an individual's death. The manner of death is the situation in which the death occurs and usually is limited to natural, accident, homicide, suicide, or undetermined.

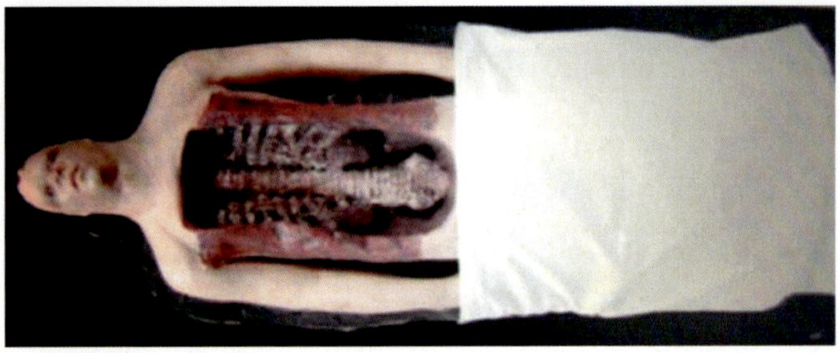

Fig. 1.7

LIST OF SELECTED MEMBER SOCIETIES OF IOFOS

- American Society of Forensic Odontology.
- Australian Society of Forensic Odontology
- British Association for Forensic Odontology
- Gemeinsamer Arbeitskreiss fur Forensische Odonto Stomatologie (Germany).
- Indian Association of Forensic Odontology
- New Zealand Society of Forensic Dentistry.
- Swedish Society of Forensic Odontology.
- The Medicolegal Society of Singapore.

LIST OF GROUPS ASSOCIATED TO IOFOS

- American Board of Forensic Odontology.
- Bangladesh Society of Forensic Odontology.
- The Croatian Group of Forensic Odontologists.
- The Hong Kong Group of Forensic Odontologists.
- The Indonesian Group of Forensic Odontologists.
- The Israeli Group of Forensic Odontologists.
- The Lithuanian Group of Forensic Odontologists.
- The Singapore Group of Forensic Odontologists.
- The Swiss Society for Forensic Medicine Odontological Section.
- The Ukraine Association of Forensic Medical Experts.
- **Forensic odontology** is the practice related to law. It can be considered as an area of specialization under dentistry as well as forensic medicine because knowledge of both the fields are vital for its activities. Although this branch appears new to us, it is probably as old as man kind itself as inscribed in the Bible. The Bible says Adam was convinced by Eve to put a 'bitemark' in an apple. But the renewed interest in this subject began in the sixties. It is an established specialty in some of the countries but in India it is still in the seminal stages.

IMPORTANCE OF DENTITION IN FORENSIC ODONTOLOGY

- The various materials used in identification of human remains are the personal belongings like pieces of clothing, jewellery, fingerprints from blood grouping and dentition. Human dentition is considered as hard tissue analogue to the fingerprints. It is almost as unique to an individual as fingerprints. Each adult human dentition consists of thirty-two teeth of which some may be missing or malformed. Effects of various environmental events, like nutrition, drugs, etc. may also be manifested on the teeth. Each race has characteristic appearances on the dentition. Then a wide variety of manipulations being done on the dentition such as restorations also add to its distinctive pattern. With such an extensive array of differences, it is extremely rare to have two similar dentitions. Apart from this, teeth are one of the most durable part of our body, which can withstand more assaults than any other part of the body. This is particularly useful in the identification of bodies in mass disasters and natural calamities. Teeth are also frequently seen in fossils.
- Forensic odontologist should have a through knowledge about the dentistry, especially the basics of anatomy including dental anatomy. He also should have an extensive knowledge of various branches of dentistry, which helps in better handling of the situations. An awareness of forensic pathology and the methods of autopsy is merited. Furthermore a comprehensive cognizance of the pertaining laws to the legal implications involved in it. So, a forensic odontologist is much more than dentist.

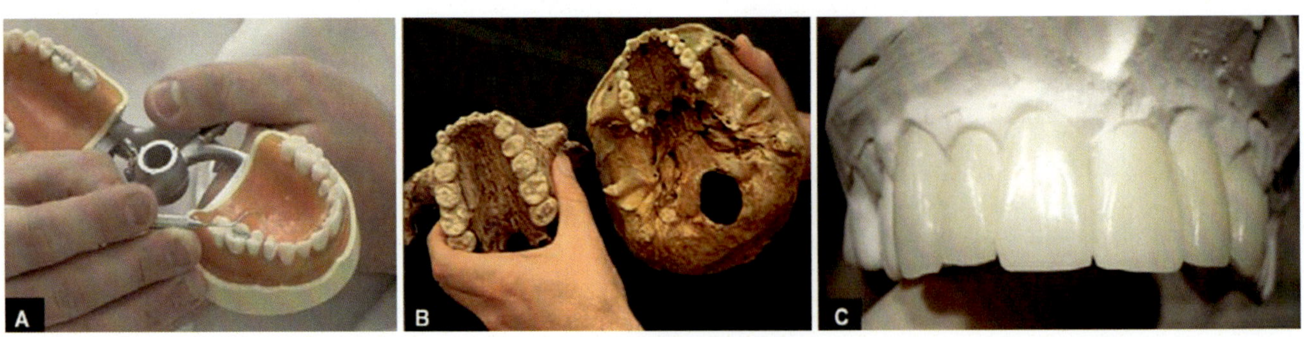

Figs 1.8A to C

FORENSIC ODONTOLOGY AREAS

Forensic odontology includes two distinct areas, **identification** and **bitemarks.**

Identification

- Identification of an individual, living or dead, is based on the theory that all individuals are unique. All humans are born with anomalies or acquired artifacts. An anomaly is a unique congenital condition (e.g. mesiodens, missing lateral incisor, hemangiomas, spinal bifida). An artifact is a man-made alteration (e.g. a dental restoration, extracted tooth, scar, tattoo, appendectomy).

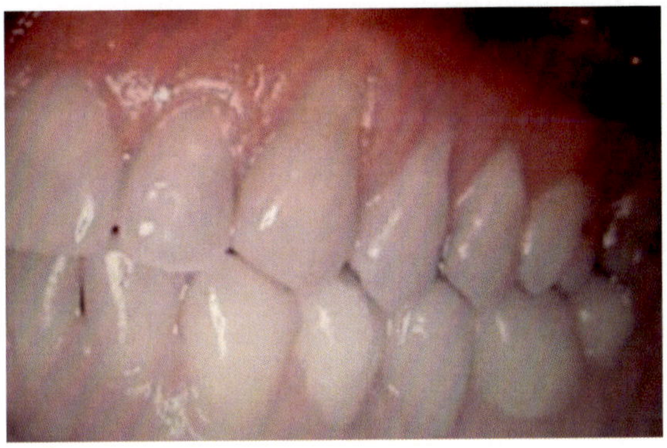

Fig. 1.9

- When an unidentified body is found, it is assumed that it could be anybody. By classifying the individual into characteristic groups (e.g. age, sex, race, height), the possibilities are narrowed. When any anomaly or artifact is found, it makes the group smaller. The more unique the characteristic, the smaller the group becomes. As more unique characteristics are noted, the comparison group becomes smaller until it reaches unity. At that point, identification can be made. An antemortem record showing these unique features must be found to match with the postmortem features of the victim.

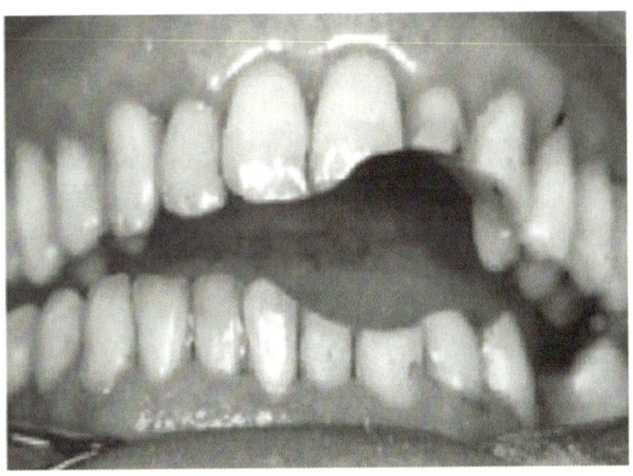

Fig. 1.10

- There are two basic types of identification, the unknown and confirmation. An unknown victim is one that has no identification on the body, and it could be almost anyone. A confirmation type of identification in one in which there is a high probability that victim may be a particular person. Forensic odontology usually is the best method to identify burned or decomposed bodies. Records of mass disasters indicate that dental identification is the most successful means of identification.

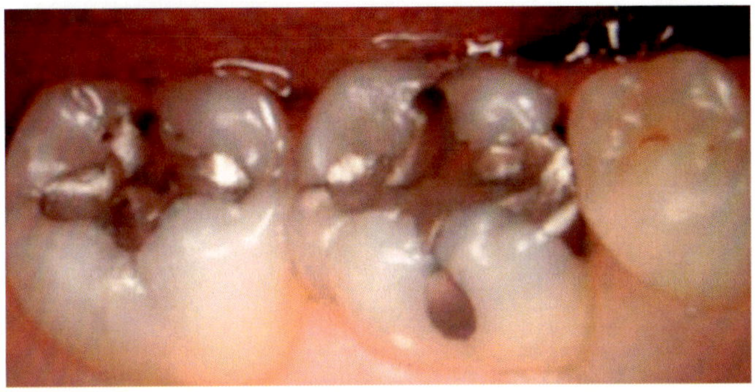

Fig. 1.11

Bitemarks

- Other distinct area of forensic odontology is bitemark identification. A pattern injury is any injury in which the instrument of injury can be determined and possibly be individualized as the weapon making the injury. A bitemark is an injury to skin in which the instruments of injury are teeth. The injury is a contusion caused by the rupture of small blood vessels as the individual teeth compress the tissue. Bitemarks

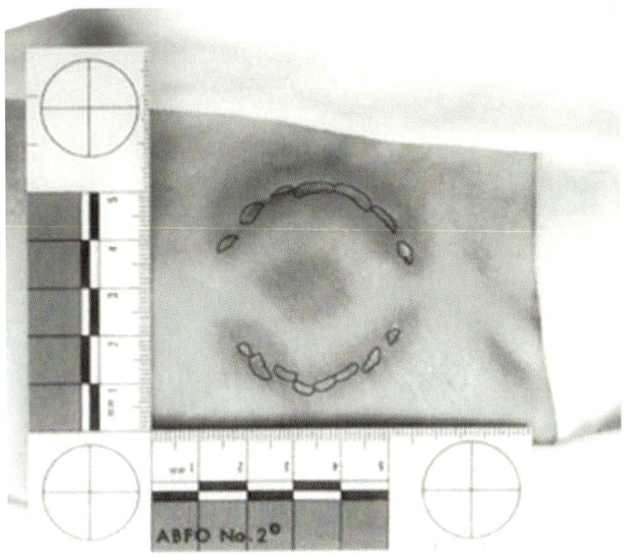

Fig. 1.12

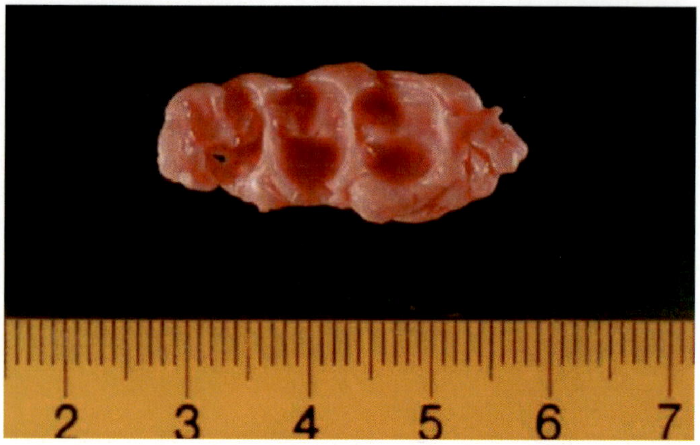

Fig. 1.13

leave blurred contusions, arrangement of the teeth is unique in every individual, and no two dentitions are identical. If the teeth leave definite marks, it should be possible to individualize them to a particular individual. Contusions tend to leak into the surrounding tissue, however, making the mark blurred or fuzzy. Despite this blurring, the forensic examiner often can narrow down the number of potential biters by excluding those who could not have made the bitemark because of definite differences (e.g. arch size, arch contour, missing teeth). By eliminating the suspects who could not have made the mark, the group of potential biters becomes small sometimes only one individual. If the suspect's bite is consistent with the bitemark, he or she may be the biter.

CHAPTER 2

Role of Dentists

ROLE OF DENTISTS IN MASS DISASTER IDENTIFICATION

- The term "mass disaster" means a chaotic event, initiated by a destructive force which results in the multiple fatalities necessitating identification. Mass disasters can be natural disasters due to earth quakes, hurricanes, fire storms and floods, accidental disasters due to fires, transportation or industrial accidents and criminal disasters such as serial homicides bombings, etc.

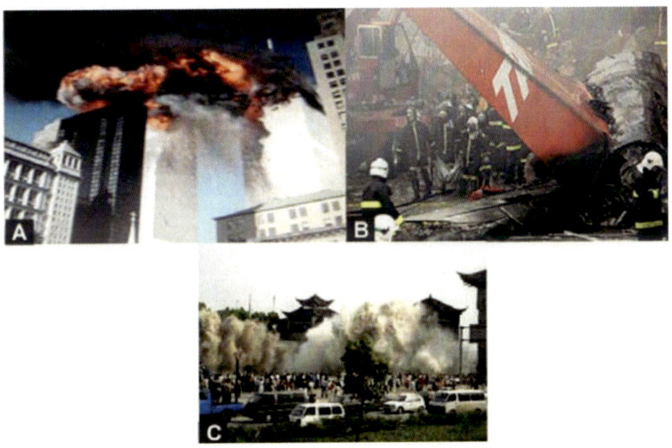

Figs 2.1A to C

- General principles of dental identification applies to mass disaster identification. But mass disasters are associated with multiple fatalities scattered throughout broad areas, may be associated with loss of antemortem records, remains may be hidden, dismembered or mutilated, proper facilities to carryout examination may not be available because most often temporary mortuary is set up in the scene of disaster causing difficulty in identification of victims. So properly trained individuals work as a team to deal with such disasters. This organized team is trained to face emergency situations.
- Mock mass disaster exercises are included in training programs. Training sessions can be used to counsel the dental team and to inform members of the post-traumatic stress often associated with this type of forensic work. This stress is a result of the sensory and psychological insults encountered by the dentist who is dealing with human death on a large scale.
- The forensic dentistry team is headed by a chief with few members. The dental team which is involved in the process of identification can be divided into home team and away team.

Home Team (Antemortem Subsection)

- Home team is responsible for the collection of antemortem data, usually this team is housed in the disaster coordinating center or near the disaster site. Before starting the actual work the team leader should brief police officers about the procedures to be followed. A prepared hand out should be given to the members of the team. Communication systems with telephones, fax machines, etc. should be established.
- All antemortem dental records including charts, radiographs, models and photographs of missing victims should be collected from dentists, hospitals and other sources. Once when the records are collected they have to be entered in a standardized antemortem data form (e.g. antemortem record chart, Interpol design). Entry should be made by at least two members of the team. All the records should be filed alphabetically.

Away Team (Postmortem Dental Examination Subsection)

- Members belonging to this team should be prepared to leave to distant places on getting information. They should be immunized against various diseases such as hepatitis B and typhoid.
- Examination of the remains is carried out by two or three members and cross-checked. Extra- and

intraoral radiographs, photographs should be taken. Dental charts must be filled accurately. While taking radiographs, necessary precautions should be taken to avoid exposing the people working in the area.

- The postmortem forms are divided into various subsections according to sex, age and types of dental treatments. When only portions of body are recovered, the forms can be kept under "unsexed" subsection. A master copy is prepared with all postmortem records in numerical order.

Comparison Methods

Comparison of ante- and postmortem records may be performed by manual method or by using computers. Use of computers reduces tedious and time consuming manual sorting of records. One of the first mass disaster where computers were used was **"Big Thompson Cayon Flood".**

Commonly used Computer Programs

- The FBI-NCIC program, based on the California Dental Identification System. CAPMI (Computer Assisted Postmortem Identification) developed by US Army Institute of Dental Research.

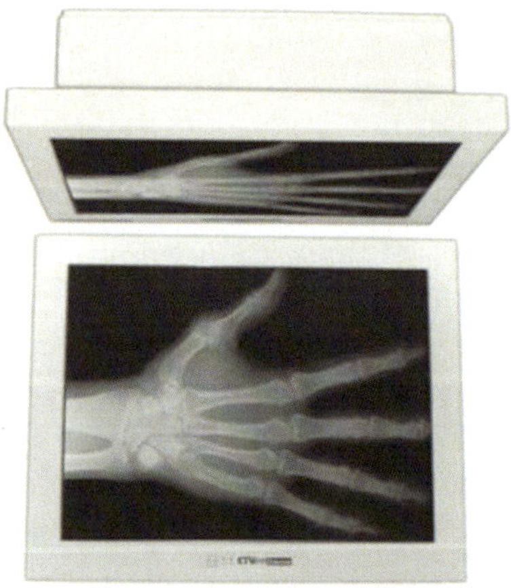

Fig. 2.2

Tooth Pics-Match Pics, developed by Class-I Inc.
Indent exe developed by McGivney J.
MUPIS system developed by Dr Bell.
Win ID developed by McGivney J.

- Computers greatly help to show records with greatest probability of containing a positive evidence, after checking all ante- and postmortem records. When utilizing computers it, is necessary to transcribe the data from dental records to the computer code form.
- The identification from dental data is the result of human thought process and computers can only aid to certain extent. Whenever possible dental

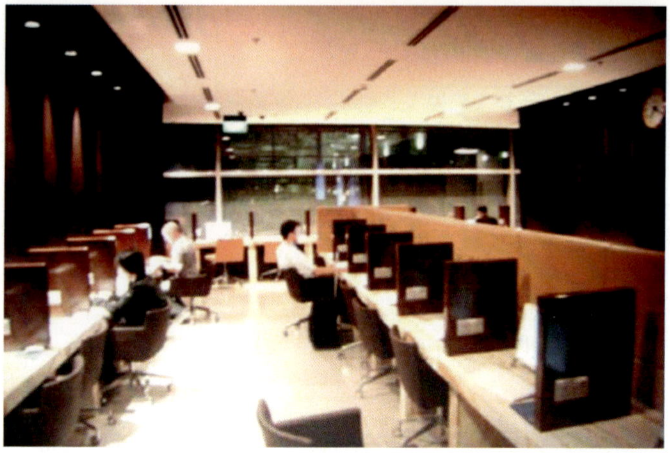

Fig. 2.3

identification should be matched with data from radiographs, fingerprints or physical features to provide a "positive identification".

Because of reasons listed below some of the remains can't be identified through dental evidence.

Inadequate or Absence of Antemortem Data

This problem is due to failure to maintain dental records by dentists, inadequate records provided by the dentists or failure to obtain name, address of the dentist who has treated the patient and patients who have not undergone any dental treatment.

Missing Persons are Foreign Nationals

Either embassy of the foreign victims or forensic dentists in their country may be contacted through International Organization for forensic odontostomatology.

Poor or Inadequate Postmortem Data

This may be due to incomplete recovery of the remains or damage to the remains beyond recognition.

Incorrect Data in the Records

Incorrect data may be entered in ante or postmortem datas. This should be reduced by repeated cross-checking of records by various members of the team and taking precautions to avoid possible mistakes during data entry into the computer.

MASS DISASTER GENETICS

A new, accurate method was used by Ballantyne in disaster victim identification by using "DNA typing". 139 out of 141 victims (98.6%) were positively identified by comparing DNA profiles obtained from human remains with those obtained from close biological relatives. Chance of mismatch between related individuals when this method is used is only one in two million.

ADVANTAGES

- DNA printing gives highly accurate positive identification.
- DNA printing may be the only means for identification of victims when there is no antemortem records.

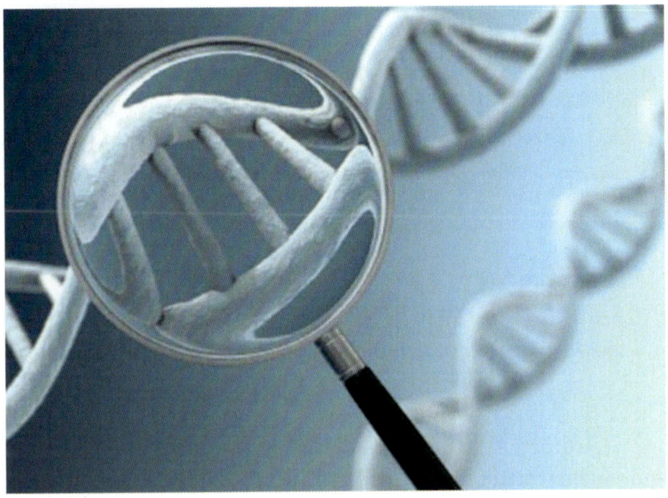

Fig. 2.4

- Teeth are used as source of DNA in many mass disaster cases for DNA fingerprinting because they resist environmental damage, easier to transport and provide high quality DNA compared to that of bone. Boles et al have described in detail regarding DNA extraction from teeth, which they have successfully applied to identify victims of 10-year-old mass graves.
- The positive identification of living or deceased persons using the unique traits and characteristics of the teeth and jaws is a cornerstone of forensic science. It is the most common way that forensic dentists (odontologists) are involved in casework, and in some instances it can be one of the most challenging aspects of the discipline. Forensic denstists can compare characteristics recorded in a patient's dental chart, usually obtained from the private dentist, with the dental characteristics found in an unknown person or a found body. If the characteristics are the same, the unknown can be identified as the person for whom the previous dental records were produced.
- The teeth are the hardest substances in the human body and may be the only method available to identify the decedent. Teeth potentially can survive most of

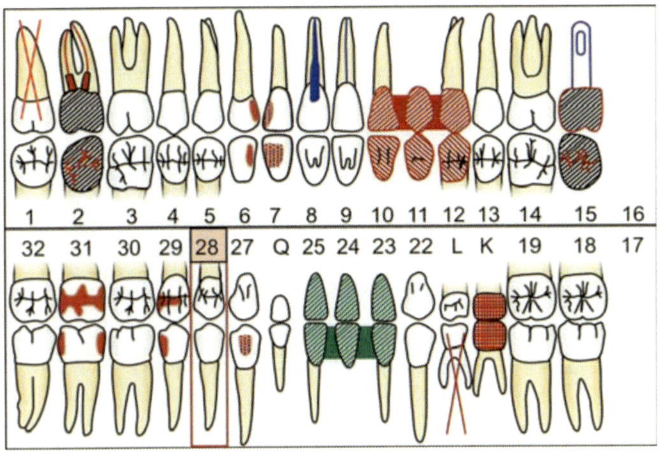

Fig. 2.5

the insults and consequences encountered at death and during decomposition. In cases in which the body is exposed to tremendous forces or extreme temperatures, such as explosive automobile or aircraft accidents, the teeth often can survive well enough to be used to identify people involved in the mishap.

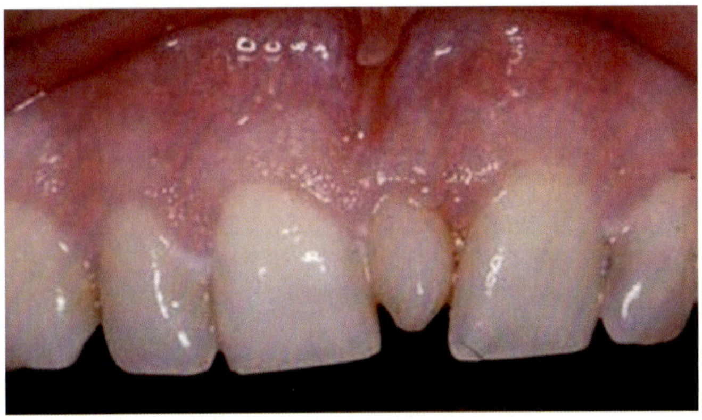

Fig. 2.6

- Currently, there are three types of personal identification circumstances that use the teeth, jaws, and orofacial characteristics. Two of these have been used for many decades and are the forensic dentist's primary responsibility.
  - The first, called comparative dental identification, involved the comparison of antemortem (before death) and postmortem (after death) dental records to determine if the body is that of the person of interest.
  - The second, called reconstructive postmortem dental profiling, is used in cases in which there is no suspicion as to who the decedent may be. Information can be gathered and provided to authorities by dentists about certain criteria, such

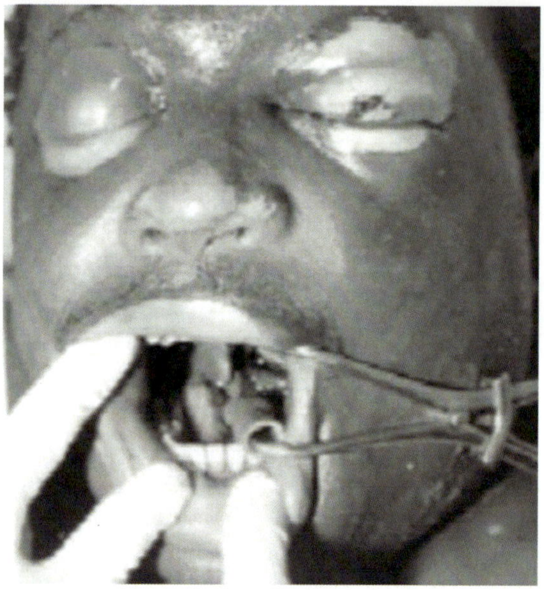

Fig. 2.7

as the age, race and sex of the decedent, to reduce the scope of the search for antemortem records of potential victims.

– The third type of dental identification, rather than relying on dental morphology or therapeutic changes, focuses on the application of modern forensic DNA profiling methods to oral tissues to establish identity. This method can be used when dental treatments or other traits from dental records are not available for comparison.

- Dentistry's role in the resolution of these cases usually occurs when the missing person has died by accident, natural causes, or homicidal violence. Although occasional cases dealing with amnesia victims are resolved with the assistance of dentistry, most cases use dentistry to aid in the identification of recovered unidentified human remains. To understand dentistry's role fully with regard to missing person cases, one first must have a basic understanding of what happens when an individual disappears and what happens when human remains are recovered. The collection of dental records is one of the easiest tasks when investigating a missing person case.
- Dental radiographs are the most common type of dental information that is collected. It is important to submit original radiographs. Sometimes identification is made using minute anatomic features, such as trabecular patterns, nutrient canals, auxiliary root canals, and sinus lining outlines. Many of these features are not clear in copied radiographs. Some states are beginning to digitize the radiographs for expedient transmission to remote locations for comparison with possible radiographic findings of found remains. Original radiographs digitize with much more detail than copies.

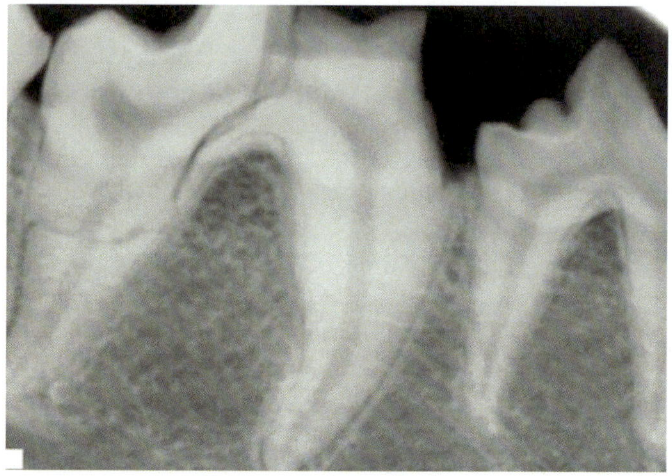

Fig. 2.8

- Bitewing radiographs often are the only types of film that are submitted because they may be most recent radiographs taken of the missing person. All films on record for the individual should be submitted to the investigating agency because older films may show different details or angles that may show identifying features that are not present on the most recent films. Panoramic, cephalometric, and tomographic radiographs show features other than the teeth that may play a crucial role in the identification of the individual.

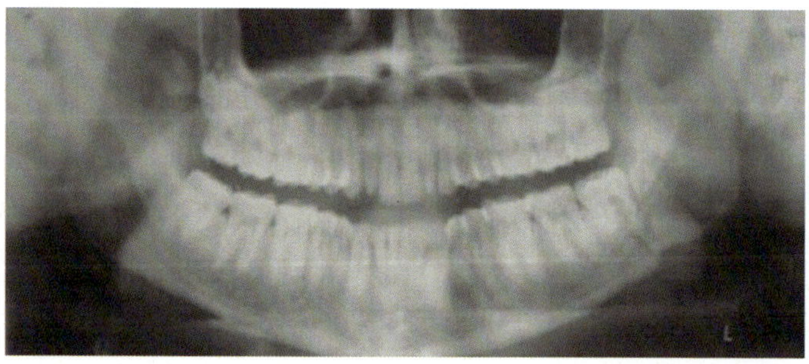

Fig. 2.9

- Written records are important in developing a complete and accurate dental profile of an individual. Radiographs usually are taken before the initiation of treatment and do not depict the most current condition of the teeth. By reviewing the written records along with the radiographs, the examining dentist can develop an accurate dental profile that allows the investigator to prioritize the list of possible identification candidates to those that correlate most closely to the dental conditions of an unidentified individual.

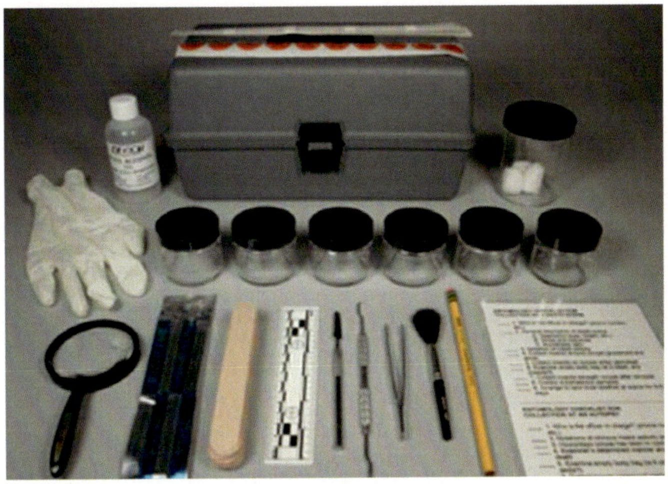

Fig. 2.10

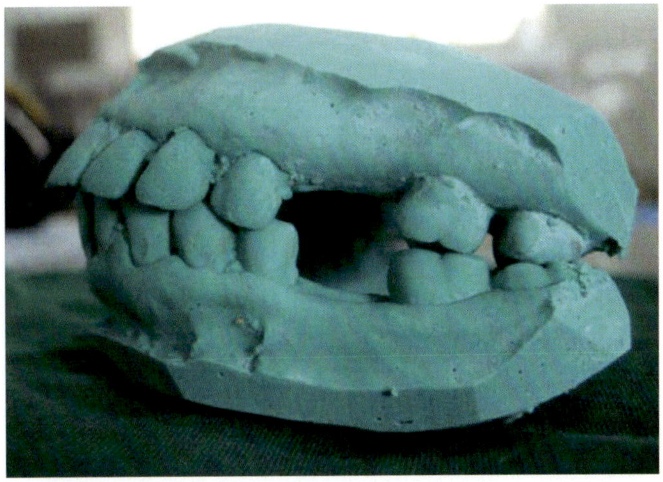

Fig. 2.11

- With the general reduction in decayed, missing, and filled teeth as a result of improved dental practices and care, anatomic information is increasingly important in the identification process. As mentioned earlier, radiographs are useful for comparison of these features; however, other dental evidence can be extremely useful. One of the easiest and clearest ways of establishing identification is by using intraoral photographs or dental models in the comparison of anatomic features to an unknown individual. The arch shape, rugae patterns, occlusal anatomy, and occlusal wear patterns are a few of the features that can be used to identify the individual. Extroral photographs can be used to perform a photographic superimposition of facial features to determine possible identifications.

DISADVANTAGES

- Cost and time taken for the DNA typing is more.
- Even though this method provides biologic relationship it may not be unique to an individual. For example, there may be other siblings of the same sex involved in the disaster. This may be overcome by recovering DNA from personal effects such as tooth brush instead of DNA from close biologic relatives from matching.

CHAPTER 3

Dental Identification

MEANS OF IDENTIFICATION

- Identification of human remains is established by several means probably the most common method is a visual identification. If the remains are viewable, family or friends of the deceased can attest to their identity because viewing is not always possible because of the cause of death or the death interval (the amount of time that occurs between the actual time of death and the time at which the remains are discovered). Extensive trauma, burns, and decomposition do not allow for a visual confirmation of the identification. When these circumstances are present, other means of identification must be used.

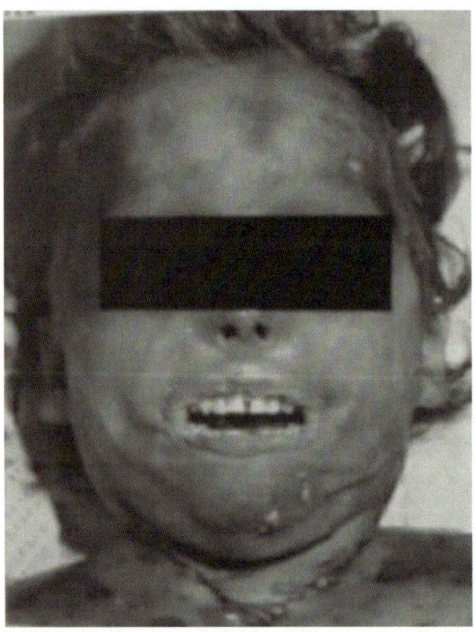

Fig. 3.1

- Fingerprints commonly are used for identification. Huge databases of fingerprints are available for comparison with fingerprints that are available from recovered human remains. Most of these databases contain fingerprints of individuals that have been handled by the law enforcement community.

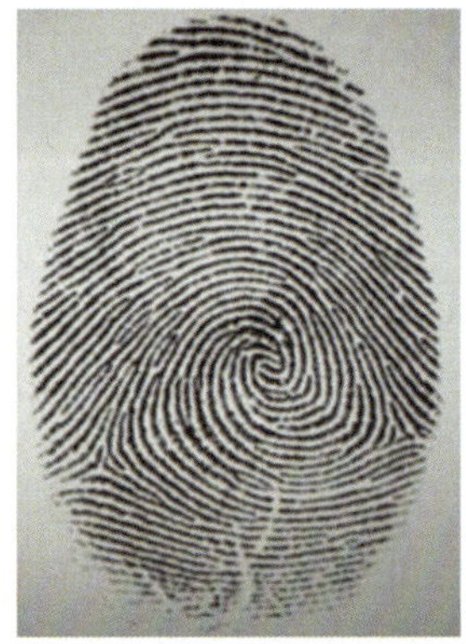

Fig. 3.2

- The emerging science of DNA matching is useful for identification, but databases for comparison are limited at this time. The Military and the Law Enforcement Communities are establishing database of DNA information for service people and sex offenders. DNA has been useful in the identification process when all other sources of identification have been exhausted. DNA matching usually requires that the Investigating Agency has some idea of the identity of the remains. Reference samples are taken from the family of the suspected deceased, then compared with DNA samples taken fom the recovered remains.

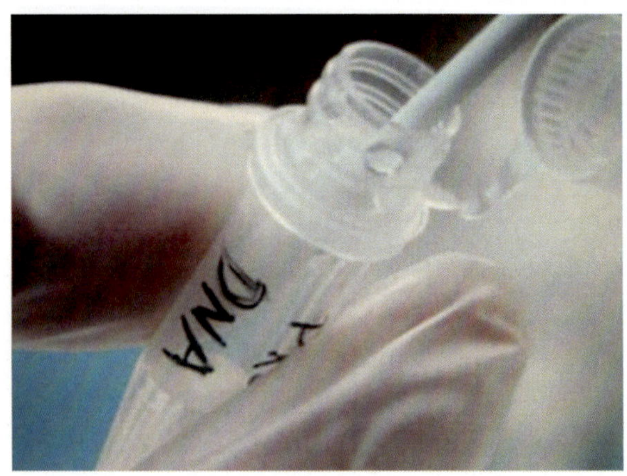

Fig. 3.3

Dental Identification

- Dental identification is common in the establishment of the identity of recovered human remains. The establishment of a dental identification requires the collection of dental information from the recovered remains. Once this information has been completed, a comparison of this information is made with the dental information of the missing or suspected individual collected from the last dentist of record. In most cases, the identity of the individual is suspected because of circumstances surrounding the recovery of the remains. Car and aircraft accidents, house fires, and other incidents in which the identity of the occupants is suspected is confirmed using dental data. Personal items that are found with the body give the investigator clues as to the possible identity of the individual. Most jurisdiction require scientific confirmation of identity, and this, as noted previously, usually is accomplished thorough fingerprints, dentition, or DNA.
- The role of the dentist in this part of the missing persons case is in evidence collection. The dental information should be collected from the remains as accurately and completely as possible. This process includes a visual examination of the oral structures, noting any features that may aid in the identification, such as tori, endodontics treatment, dental implants or other surgical appliances, and other unusual anatomic features, as well as the complete charting of existing restorations.

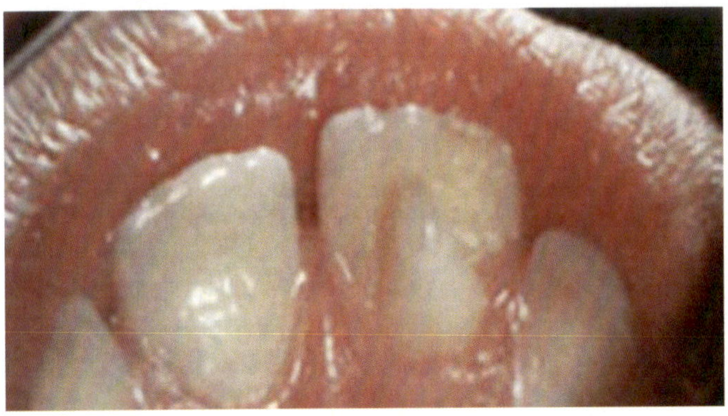

Fig. 3.4

- Photographs of the deceased individual should be taken for two reasons. The first reason is to show the condition of the remains before and after the examination process. Access to the oral structures for a visual and radiographic examination frequently requires some tissue manipulation or, in rare cases, complete resection of the maxillary and mandibular arches. Justification for these procedures can be documented easily in photographs. Intraoral photographs of the deceased also can be used to establish identity, especially if the individual had undergone orthodontic treatment and the treatment photographs are available from the orthodontist record.

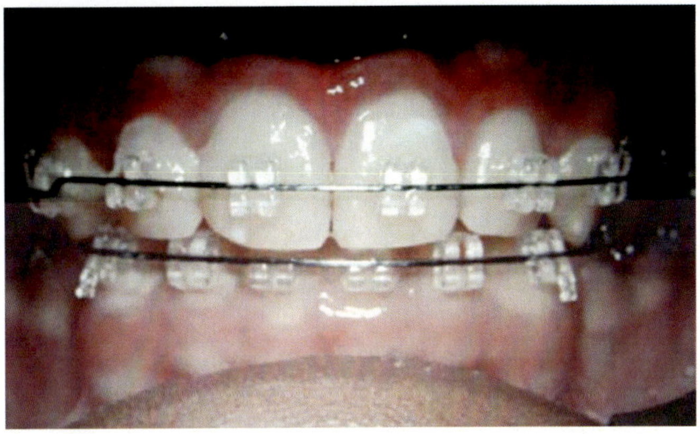

Fig. 3.5

- Impressions of the deceased's dentition can be important in the identification process. Orthodontists and restorative dentists often take impressions of the dentition to document or fabricate restorative and treatment appliances. These models, when available, can provide a vast amount of identification information by adding a three-dimensional factor to the comparison process that the two-dimensional radiographs cannot demonstrate. The dentist's involvement in the collection of dental information regarding the deceased individual requires all the skills and experience that the dentist has gained from the treatment of patients.

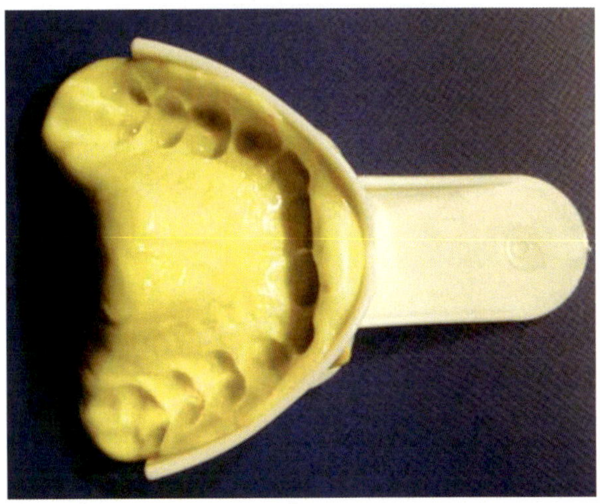

Fig. 3.6

- The most common role of the forensic dentist is the identification of deceased individuals. Dental identification takes two main forms.

- Firstly, the most frequently performed examination is a comparative identification that is used to establish (to a high degree of certainty) that the remains of a decedent and a person represented by antemortem (before death) dental records are of the same individual. Information from the body or circumstances usually contains clues as to who has died.

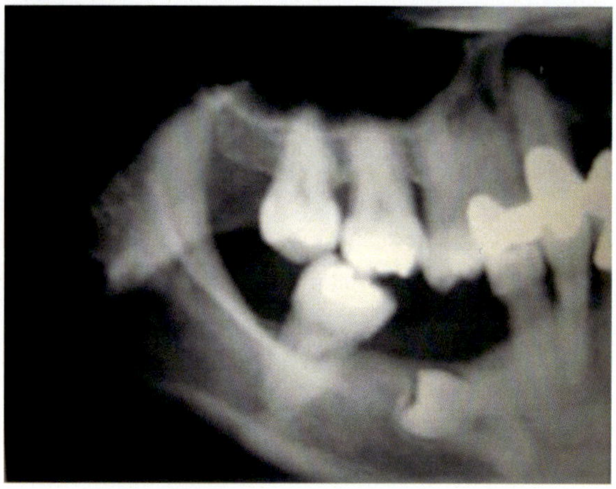

Fig. 3.7

- Secondly, in those cases where antemortem records are not available, and no clues to the possible identity exist, a postmortem (after death) dental profile is completed by the forensic dentist suggesting characteristics of the individual likely to narrow the search for the antemortem materials.

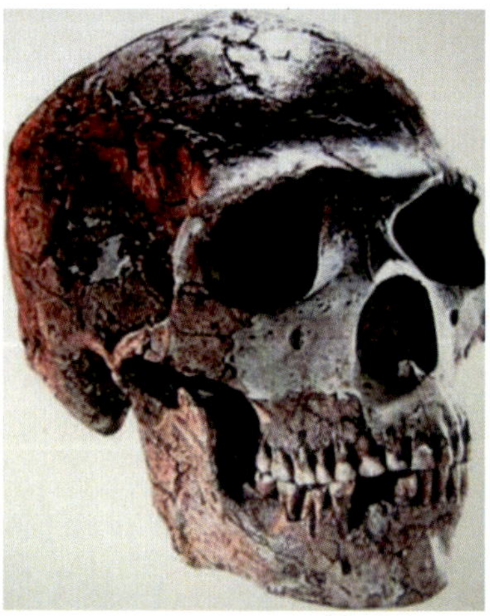

Fig. 3.8

- Dental identification of humans occurs for a number of different reasons and in a number of different situations. The bodies of victims of violent crimes, fires, motor vehicle accidents and workplace accidents, can be disfigured to such an extent that identification by a family member is neither reliable nor desirable. Persons who have been deceased for some time prior to discovery and those found in water also present unpleasant and difficult visual identifications. Dental identifications have always played a key role in natural and man made disaster situations and in particular the mass casualties normally associated with aviation disasters. Because of the lack of a comprehensive fingerprint database, dental identification continues to be crucial.

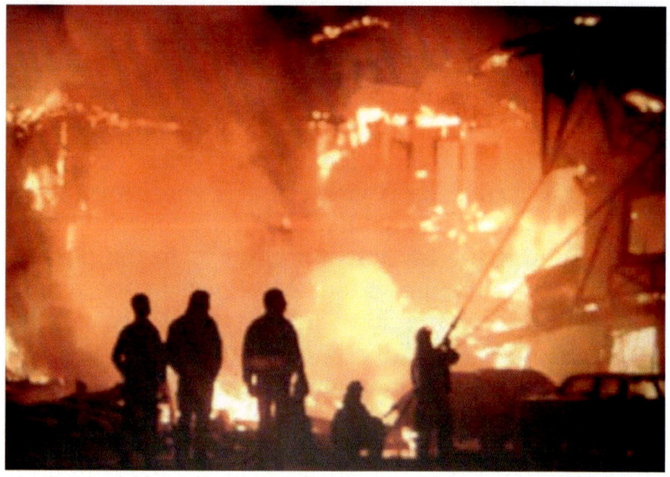

Fig. 3.9

Comparative Dental Identification

- The central dogma of dental identification is that postmortem dental remains can be compared with antemortem dental records, including written notes, study casts, radiographs, etc. to confirm identity. Clearly, individuals with numerous and complex dental treatments are often easier to identify than those individuals with little or no restorative treatment. The teeth not only represent a suitable repository for such unique and identifying features, they also survive most postmortem events that can disrupt or change other body tissues. A presumptive or tentative identification is available (i.e. wallet or driving licence may be found on the body) and this will enable antemortem records to be located. In other instances, the geographical location in which the body is found or other physical characteristics and circumstantial evidence, may enable a putative identification to be made, frequently using data from the missing persons database. Antemortem records are then obtained from the dentist of record.
- The forensic dentist produces the postmortem record by careful charting and written descriptions of the dental structures and radiographs. If the antemortem records are available at this time, postmortem radiographs should be taken to replicate the type and angle of these. Radiographs should be marked with a

rubber-dam punch to indicate antemortem and postmortem to prevent confusion — one hole for antemortem films and two holes for postmortem films. Once the postmortem record is complete, a comparison between the two records can be carried out. A methodical and systematic comparison is required, examining each tooth and surrounding structures in turn. While dental restoration figure significantly in the identification process, many other oral features are assessed. Additional features play an increasingly important role in those individuals with minimal restorations. Because of the progressive decrease in dental caries, so-called non-restorative cases are likely to become more common. Similarities and discrepancies should be noted during the comparison process. There are two types of discrepancy, those that can be explained and those that cannot. Explainable discrepancies normally relate to the time elapsed between the antemortem and postmortem records. Examples include teeth extracted or restorations placed or enlarged (i.e. MO amalgam that is now MOD). If a discrepancy is unexplainable, for example a tooth is not present on the antemortem record but is present on the postmortem record then an exclusion must be made.

- A range of conclusions can be reached when reporting a dental identification. The American Board of Forensic Odontology recommends that these be limited to the following four conclusions. Positive identification : The antemortem and postmortem data match in sufficient detail, with no unexplainable discrepancies, to establish that they are from the same individual. Possible identification : The antemortem and postmortem data have consistent features but, because of the quality of either the postmortem remains or the antemortem evidence, it is not possible to establish identity positively.
- **Insufficient evidence:** The available information is insufficient to form the basis for a conclusion. Exclusion : The antemortem and postmortem data are clearly inconsistent.
- It is important to note that there is no minimum number of concordant points or features that are required for a positive identification. In many cases, a single tooth can be used for identification if it contains sufficient unique features. Equally, a full-mouth series of radiographs may not reveal sufficient detail to render a positive conclusion. The discretion of identification lies with the odontologist who must be prepared to justify the conclusions in court, surely the ultimate in peer- review. When antemortem dental records are unavailable and other methods of identification are not possible, the forensic dentist can assist in limiting the population pool to which the deceased is likely to belong and thus increase the likelyhood of locating antemortem dental records. This process is known as postmortem dental profiling. The information from this process will enable a more focused search for antemortem records. A post-mortem dental profile will typically provide information on the deceased; age, ancestry back-ground, sex and socioeconomic status. In some instances it is possible to provide additional information regarding occupation, dietary habits, habitual behavior and occasionally on dental or systemic diseases.

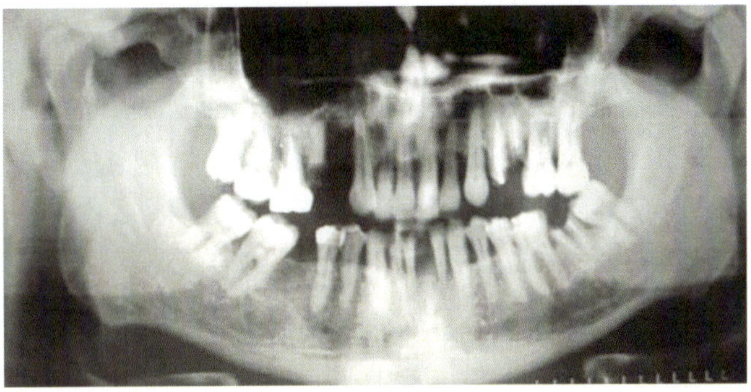

Fig. 3.10

- Forensic anthropologists most often provide details of osteological studies, but forensic dentists can assist in the process. The determination of sex and ancestry can be assessed from skull shape and form. Generally, from skull appearance, forensic dentists can determine race. Additional characteristics, such as cusps of Carabelli, shovel- shaped incisors and multi-cusped premolars, can also assist in determiniation of ancestry. Sex determination is usually based on cranial appearance, as no sex differences are apparent in the morphology of teeth. Microscopic examination of teeth can confirm sex by the presence or absence of Y-chromatin and DNA analysis can also reveal sex.

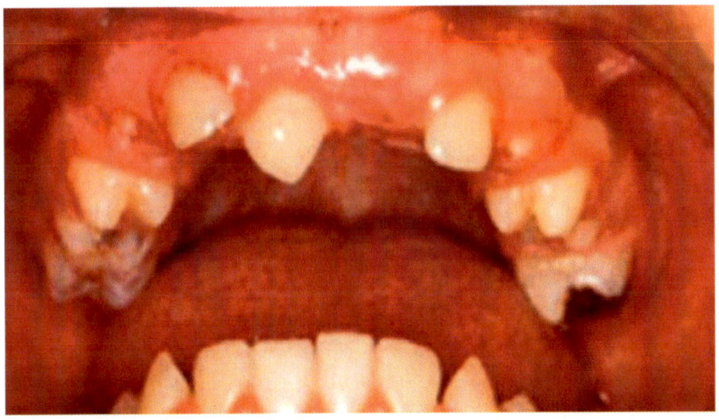

Fig. 3.11

- Dental structures can provide useful indicators to the individual's chronological age. The age of children (including fetuses and neonates) can be determined by the analysis of tooth development and subsequent comparison with developmental charts. Charts such as those developed by Ubelaker graphically illustrate the development of the dentition from 5 months *in utero* to 35 years, illustrating the deciduous, mixed and permanent dentitions. It is important to note that when determining sub-adult ages, eruption dates of the teeth are highly variable and the actual developmental stages of the teeth are more accurate. Third molar development is used by some forensic dentists to assign age to young adults although doubts concerning the accuracy of this technique will be raised by the practitioner's own experience of the variability of these teeth. Periodontal disease progression, excessive wear, multiple restorations, extractions, bone pathosis and complex restorative work may indicate an older individual. Some odontologists advocate the use of aspartic acid recemization. Additional methods include the use of SEM-EDXA, a method used to examine dentine in relation to age determination. A recent study examined the use of root length in the determination of age in pediatric cases.

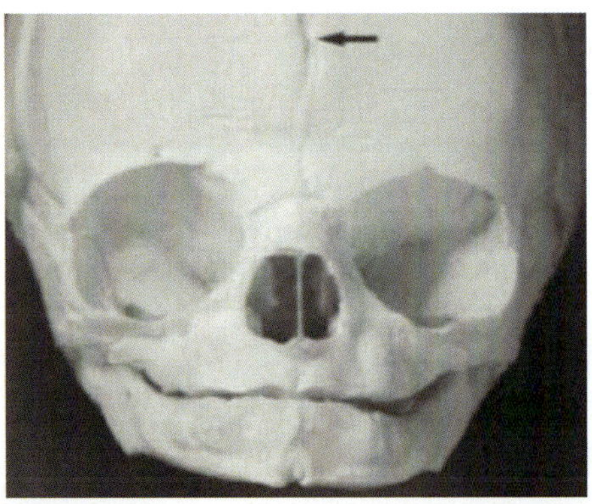

Fig. 3.12

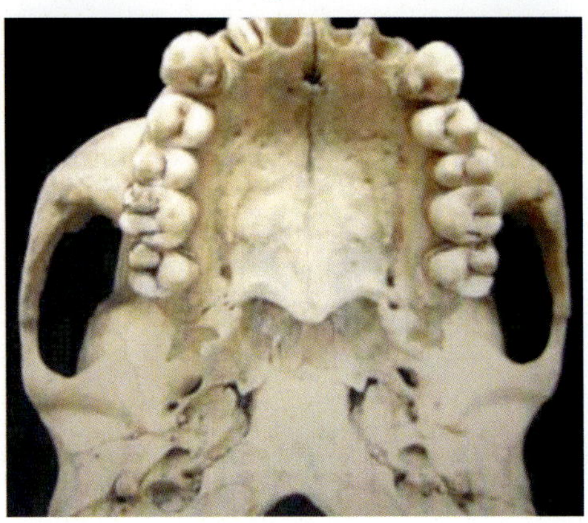

Fig. 3.13

- The presence of erosion can suggest alcohol or substance abuse, an eating disorder or even hiatus hernia while stains can indicate smoking, tetracycline use or betel-nut chewing. Unusual wear patterns may result from pipe stems, cigarette holders, hairpins, carpet tacks or previous orthodontic treatment. The quality, quantity and presence or absence of dental treatment may give an indication of socioeconomic status or likely country of residence. If the postmortem profile does not elicit the tentative identity of the deceased it may be necessary to reconstruct the individual's appearance during life. This is the responsibility of forensic artists who use the dental profile to help with the facial reproduction.

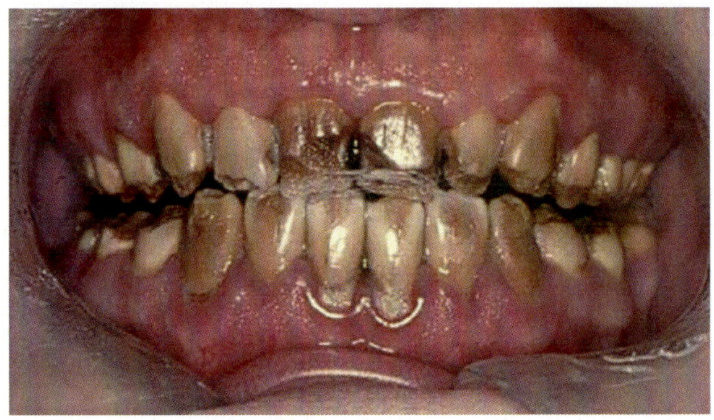

Fig. 3.14

Other Methods of Dental Identification

- The two processes described above, comparative identification and postmortem profiling, represent the most common methods of dental identification. However, in some instances more novel and innovative techniques have been applied. There have been a number of requests from individuals and dental organizations over the year to insist that dental prothesis are labeled with the patient's name or a unique number. Labeled dentures can be of great assistance in the identification of individuals.

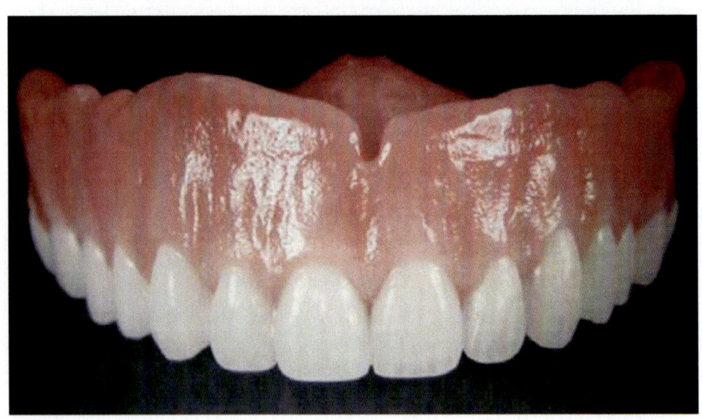

Fig. 3.15

- Unlabeled dentures have been recovered from patients and then fitted to casts retained by the treating dentist or laboratory, and this has been an accepted method of identification. Other dental appliances, such as removable orthodontic braces have also been used for identification purposes. The use of palatal rugae patterns rendered on dental casts to compare with found remains. Positive identification have resulted from this technique.

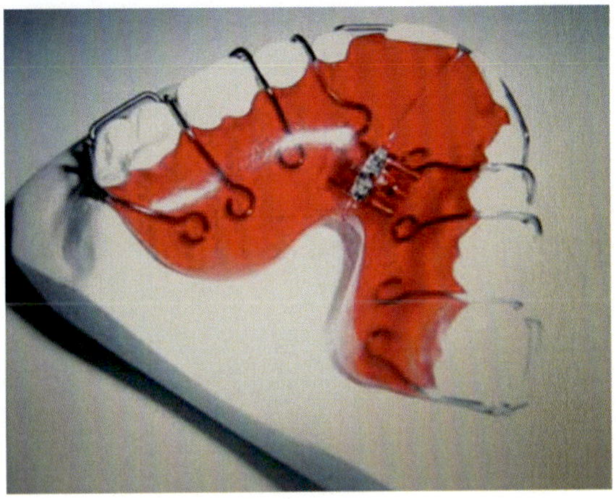

Fig. 3.16

- Dental materials have provided clues to assist identification. SEM-EDX has been used to identify the composition of a glass-ionomer restoration and then traced this back to a prison where the filling was placed. Dental records secured the identification of the individual. It was possible to identify Kevlar fibers that had been placed within a lower denture to reinforce it. This rare procedure enabled an identification of the wearer who was a victim of homicide.

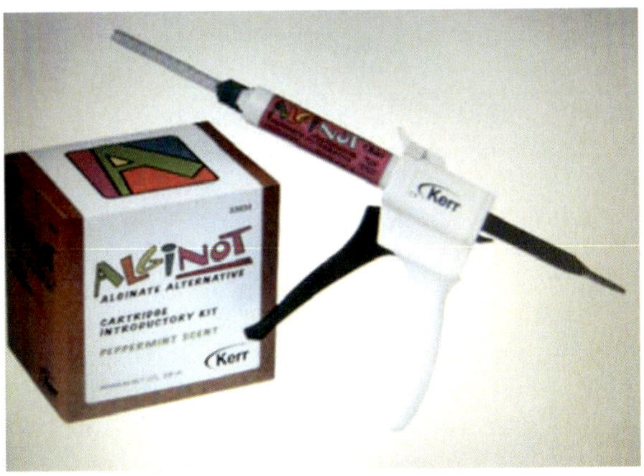

Fig. 3.17

- Because of the resistant nature of dental tissues to environmental assaults, such as incineration, immersion, trauma, mutilation and decomposition, teeth represent an excellent source of DNA material. When conventional dental identification methods fails, this biological material can provide the necessary link to prove identity. With the advent of the polymerase chain reaction (PCR), a technique that allows amplification of DNA at pre-selected, specific sites, this source of evidence is becoming increasingly popular with investigators. Comparison of DNA preserved in and extracted from the teeth of an unidentified individual can be made to a known antemortem sample (stored blood, hairbrush, clothing, cervical smear, biopsy, etc.) or to a parent or sibling.

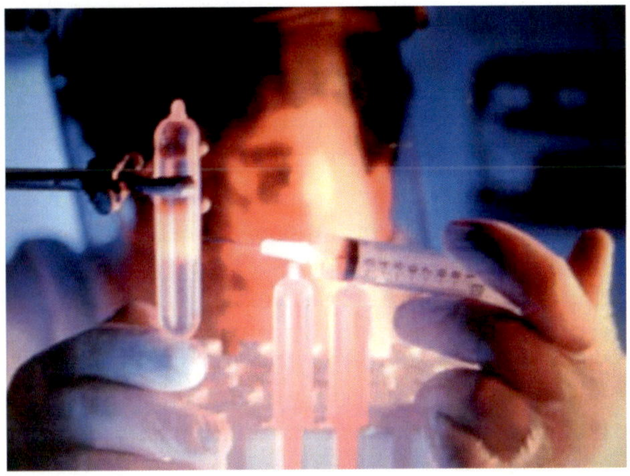

Fig. 3.18

- Genomic DNA is found in the nucleus of each cell and represents the DNA source for most forensic applications, (there are no nuclei, and hence there is no DNA, in red blood cells). When body tissues have decomposed, the structures of the enamel, dentine and pulp complex persist. It is necessary to extract the DNA from the calcified tissues. The cryogenic grinding method is employed. Teeth represent an excellent source of genomic DNA. Indeed, the authors have found that even root-filled teeth supply sufficient biological material for PCR analysis.

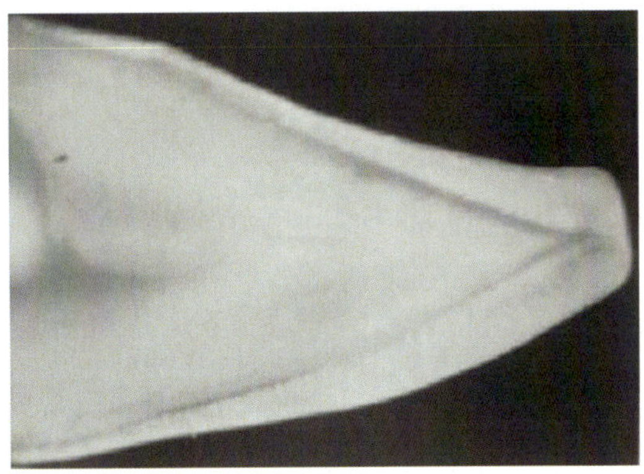

Fig. 3.19

PCR-based analysis produces a DNA profile that can be compared with known antemortem samples or paternal DNA. The identification of individuals is not the only use for dental DNA. The technique has allowed criminal investigators to link victims to crime scenes once the body has been removed and incinerated.

- In addition to genomic DNA, cells contain mitochondrial DNA (mtDNA), the sequence of building blocks of which can be determined to assist in identification. The main advantage of mtDNA is that there is a high copy number in each cell caused by the high number of mitochondria present in most cells. This infers that in cases where genomic DNA cannot be analyzed, possibly because it is too degraded, mtDNA may be present in sufficient quantity. In addition to its higher copy number, mtDNA is maternally inherited. This maternal inheritance pattern confers the same mtDNA sequence, barring mutations, upon siblings and all their maternal relatives. This has important implications for the identification of individuals for which there is no antemortem comparison sample. Although mitochondrial DNA is still in its infancy in forensic casework, it is a powerful technique that is likely to become commonplace in the future.

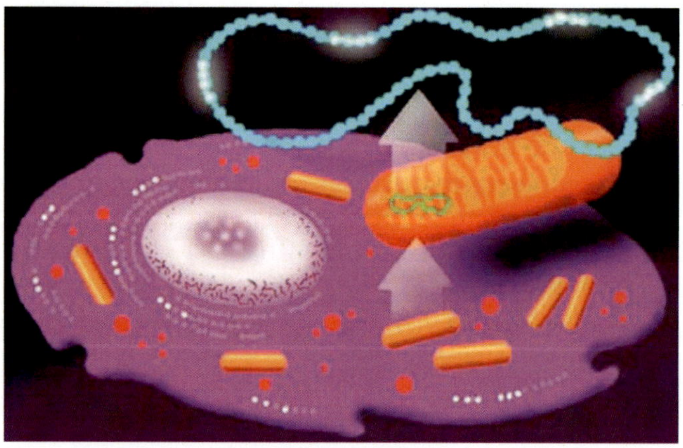

Fig. 3.20

IDENTIFICATION PROCESS

Importance of Timely Identification

How important is the timely identification of unknown human remains? Incases involving a death, little progress will be made without first establishing the true identity of the deceased. It is a well understood axiom in law enforcement that "if you can't identify the body, you can't solve the case." But there is an even more compelling, humanitarian reason for accurate and quick identifications.

Scientific Identification

- There currently exists four general methods to identify deceased human remains. They are visual recognition, fingerprint comparison, DNA analysis, and medical/dental comparison.

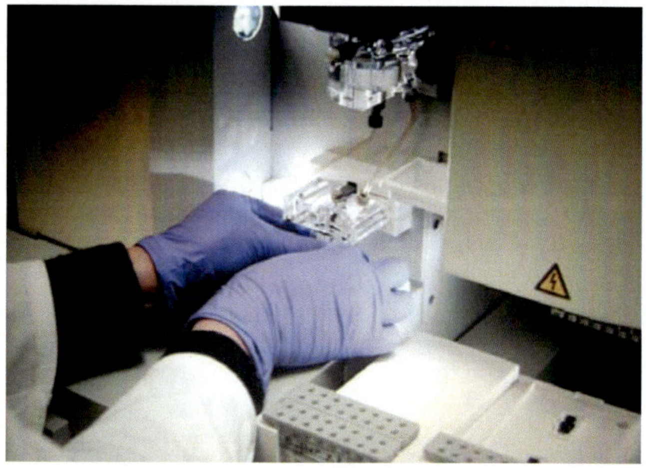

Fig. 3.21

- They all involve the direct comparison of substantive material evidence. Finger print records made or latent prints left before death can be compared to those taken from a body; DNA evidence, available before death, can be compared to that recovered from postmortem tissues;and dental and medical characteristics, discovered visually and/or via radiographs (X-rays), can be compared to antemortem records and films. There has to be a comparison of antemortem and postmortem evidence to establish a positive identification.
- All are dependent on the existence of antemortem material. The conclusions drawn by the forensic experts are only as good as the evidence with which they have to work. More than one case has been the introduction or the attempt to introduce fraudulent evidence. The prudent investigator will question the authenticity of the antemortem evidence, and do everything possible to insure its validity. In the same vein, it is equally important to document the postmortem evidence and to protect the chain of custody of that material.
- Fingerprints. when available, are generally recognized as the best form of identification. If the deceased has useable fingerprints and if they are on record some where, that comparison alone can establish positive identification. Unfortunately, it is

also a fact that today fewer people have fingerprint records taken and retained than in previous times. And women historically have been less likely to have had fingerprint records taken. In addition, fingerprints, though constant during a person's life, will start to deteriorate immediately after death as the body decomposes.

- DNA analysis has rapidly proven itself to be a valuable tool in the identification process. In addition to its value in criminal cases, it has revolutionized civil proceedings involving paternity and maternity. However, a positive identification using this technique, like the others, requires that some proven antemortem genetic material from that individual be available. Comparisons to relative, parents, siblings, etc. cannot be conclusive. These can only prove relationships, not positive identification.

Dental Identification

- The comparison of a missing person's **dental records, models and radiographs** (X-rays) with the dental evidence from unknown human remains, has **long been recognized** as one of the most reliable means of positive scientific identification. Though an individual's dental characteristics will often change during life (cavities, fillings, extractions, etc.), changes after death are very slow. In fact, the dental condition at death has been shown to last in some cases for centuries. When there is an alteration in an individual's dental condition, that change is in one direction.
- "The direction of change of status of a tooth is fixed; that is a tooth cannot have a filling on a surface and then proceed to a state in which there is filling on that surface. It can only go from having no filling on a surface to a state in which there is one." Likewise, once a tooth is extracted or otherwise missing, it cannot subsequently be present. This unidirectional change is significant during the verification process and must be considered during any comparison/ search process.
- The consulting forensic odontologist will evaluate and compare the two dental records, the postmortem and the antemortem material. It is his/her task to determine if the two records were made or could have been made from the same individual. In the end however, for there to be a positive match all inconsistencies within the written records must be explained and distinguishing features must be demonstrable in the hard material evidence, i.e. X-rays, stone models, photographs, etc.

Search/Comparison Process

- The accurate and scientific identification of an unknown human body can only be accomplished when there is a record to compare with the postmortem evidence. To be able to find that antemortem record, there has to be something to suggest that individual's possible identity. This is usually provided by some personal effect or clue found on or in the general vicinity of the body. When there are no such clues, law enforcement must use the actual physical characteristics of the victim and compare to available missing person records. For practical purposes these general physical descriptors (height, weight, eye and hair color, etc.) can be of some assistance in narrowing the field of possible identities; however, they are subject to change and are often subjective assessments. Considering the large number of missing persons in this country, this type of evidence, though important, has a limited value in an actual identification. In addition, with the passage of time many of these characteristics are lost to decomposition, skeletonization and scattering.

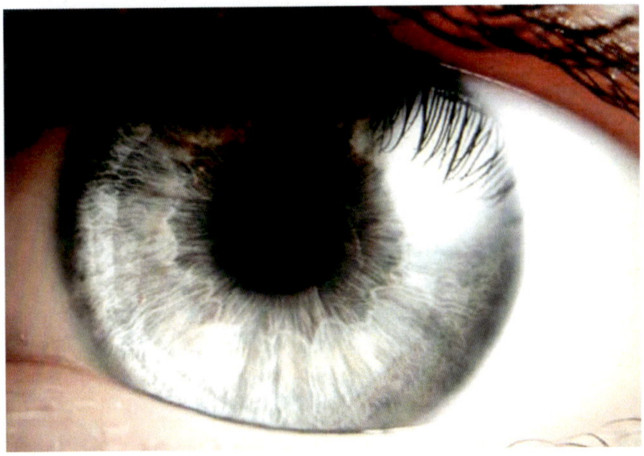

Fig. 3.22

- However, without some clue to the possible identity, no direct comparison could be accomplished. And those clues were usually non-dental in nature, i.e. personal effects, witnesses accounts, circumstances, auto registrations, etc. Additionally, in more than a few instances the dental information from unidentified bodies was not recorded for later comparison because no putative identification was discovered at the time. As a result, that information was frequently lost forever, making future comparisons impossible.
- Like fingerprints, the dental information available can provide enough individual characteristics to be

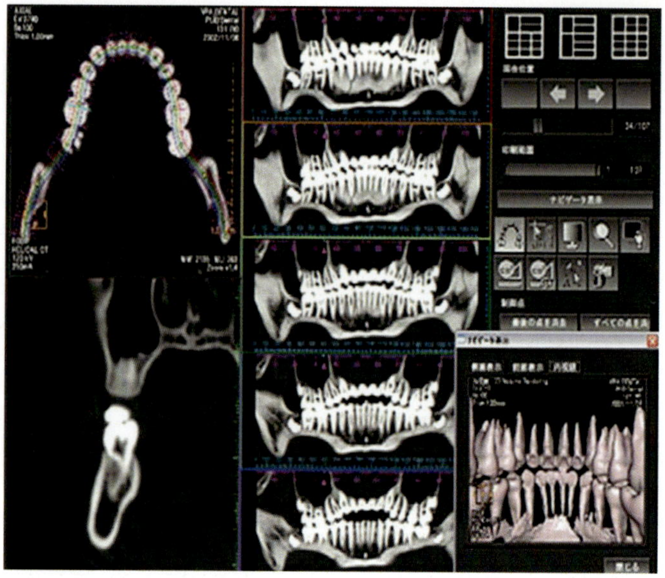

Fig. 3.23

utilized during the narrowing process. There are enough different possible combinations of variables in the human dentition, (over 8 trillion), that these alone can be used as a means to sort through to a possible (putative) identity. Taking the same methods used in a mass disaster identification operation, Jones relates them to the missing/unidentified person scenario. "To use dental data successfully for identification in those cases where non-dental clues are not available, certain procedures have to be employed... three processes must be followed: Data gathering, data comparison/selection, and final verification."

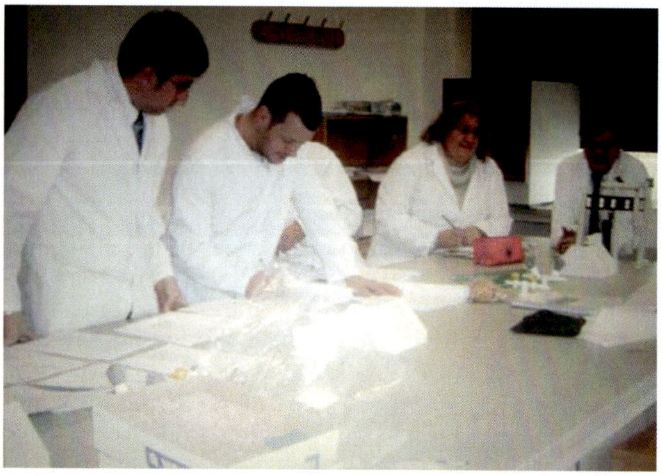

Fig. 3.24

- With the development of computer software programs designed to search and compare dental records, in a way somewhat similar to the way that Automated Fingerprint Identification System (AFIS) searches fingerprint records, it has become possible to use the dental evidence available in these types of cases as the sole vehicle to actually narrow the field of records to check. This process is called the comparison/search process. Too few agencies are taking advantage of the new technologies available. They begin by failing to gather the dental data, especially in missing persons cases. Dental information is not being routinely included in missing person reports. They also too frequently fail to record and preserve the dental evidence from unidentified bodies. The unidentified entries with dental information are at only slightly over 50%. It is clear that law enforcement needs to recognize and embrace this valuable tool in its missing and unidentified person cases.

MISSING PERSON CASES

Missing Person Report

- The missing person report begins with the first contact from a family member or friend. This is the most critical time in the entire process, and the most often neglected by police agencies. Often times the assignment to "missing persons" is either neglected or given to the most Junior Officer in the Department with turnover commonly frequent. This makes it a seemingly unimportant duty, one that no one would want to have. It may not be illegal to be missing, but these cases are important to family members and without this information some cases will go unresolved. It is important and the assignment of personnel to this task should acknowledge that importance within the department.
- It is during this initial contact that three things can be accomplished. Complete information regarding the missing needs to be recorded; the family needs to be reassured that their case is important and favorable public relations for the agency within the community should be realized. This is the time to gather as much information as possible.
- Most law enforcement agencies have standard forms for recording missing person reports. It is important that these forms include adequate space for medical and dental information. Ask the reporting person about the missing person's medical and dental history:
  - Name and address of dentist(s)
  - Did he/she go to the dentist regularly?
  - Did he/she have a regular dentist? Here? Previous home locations? Previous military service? which branch?

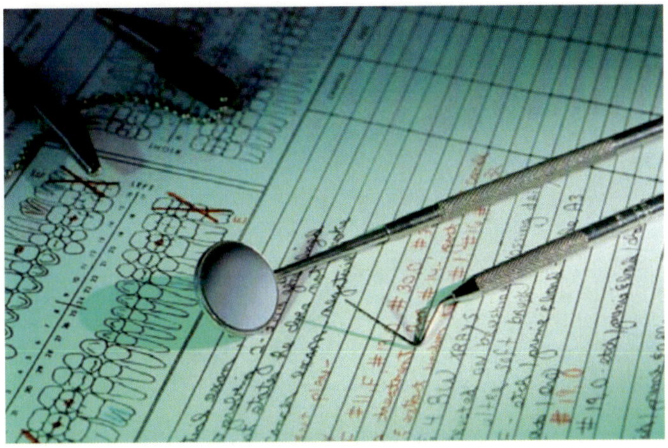

Fig. 3.25

- Other dental sources (specialists): Orthodontists (straightening), oral surgeons, periodontists (gum disease), endodontists (root canals), prosthodontists (dentures, partials, crown and bridge and implants).

- Medical history, including physician names, hospitalizations, accidents, illnesses, etc. Be specific about head and chest injuries, these often result in medical X-rays that show some dental features.

Gathering the Dental Information

- There is no real need to delay collecting the dental information beyond thirty days. This should be viewed as a maximum time for gathering and reporting. In most cases, two to three weeks are more appropriate.
- When contacting a Dental or Medical Office, the Officer should appropriately identify himself/herself and explain the nature of the investigation and the information that he/she is requesting. Most offices will voluntarily cooperate fully; some states have laws that permit police access; and if not, a subpena or threat of a subpena, will usually facilitate access. Remember, this office may have information that could lead to other sources, i.e. previous dentists, specialist referrals, medical history, etc.

All available information should be retrieved. This will include:

- Complete written records or good quality, readable photocopies. The originals are preferred.
- Original radiographs or good quality duplicates. Again the originals are preferred. If duplicates are provided they need to be accurately labeled as to left - right orientation, and include all dates, etc.
- Plaster or stone models (study models), if available.
- Photographs, if available. Some offices have prints or videos of patients in various stages of treatment.
- Any other information that is available concerning that patient.
- Military records can be researched by contacting the nearest military base with the appropriate branch of service for the missing person. The Military Intelligence Office is the resource for information concerning former members.
- Try to obtain records from more than one office if possible, even if one is quite old. This will help to authenticate the antemortem evidence.

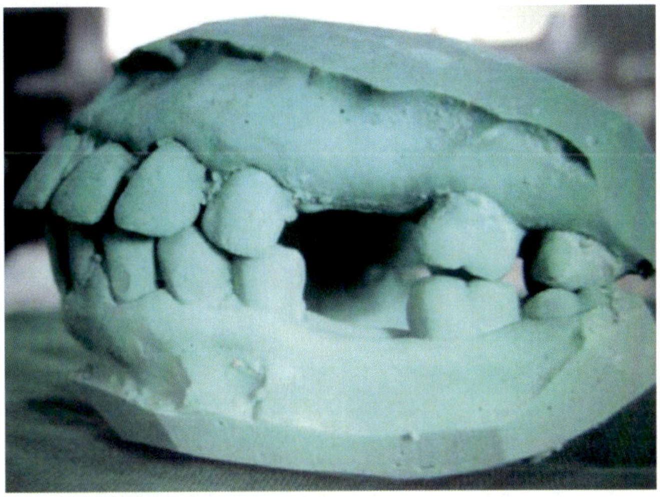

Fig. 3.26

- If no leads are available from the missing person report, contacting local area Dental Offices and Medical facilities may produce some positive results. Insurance companies and the Department of Health and Welfare may also provide useful information.
- The first thing to do after gathering this information is to include it in the missing person report. It should not just be filed away and forgotten. It has value to the case and as such it needs to be utilized. Whether a possible identity has been determined or not, the services of a forensic odontologist should be employed at this time.
- The process of deciphering and putting the dental information into a useable missing person dental form is rarely an easy task. Quite often the written dental record is incomplete or illegible. For this reason, a trained forensic dentist should be consulted for this task and the task of filling out forms from any local, state, or national dental database programs. Again, often these forms require some familiarity and experience to properly complete; and accuracy at this point is more important than speed.

- The logical first step is to have the consulting forensic expert compare this newly acquired dental data with any available postmortem evidence. If no local match is found, the information should be shared with other local, regional and national agencies that are equipped to handle this type of data.

UNIDENTIFIED BODY CASES

The dental examination is conducted under the authority and direction of the coroner/medical examiner and generally is carried out in a morgue, funeral home, or private consultant facility, as designated by each jurisdiction. A forensic odontologist should be retained to perform the examination and necessary record-taking so that all recorded information is accurate and preserved in such a way in the report as to facilitate potential comparisons. The first concern is the retrieval and transportation of the body or body parts, including the dental evidence, intact to that/those facilities.

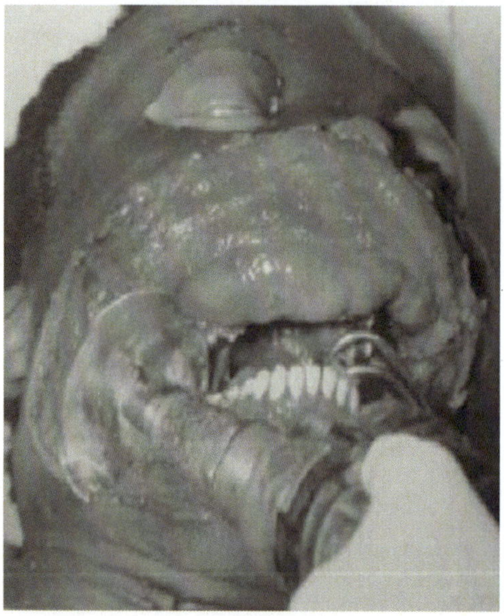

Fig. 3.27

SPECIAL CONCERNS

Severely Fragmented Body

In those cases that involve severely fragmented victims, the area should be carefully checked for any remaining and not readily apparent hard and soft tissue fragments. This may require the assistance of experts trained in fragment search and recover. Certainly, a grid search is recommended in most of these cases. Any recovered body parts or evidence should be placed ina body bag or other appropriate evidence container for transportation. It is

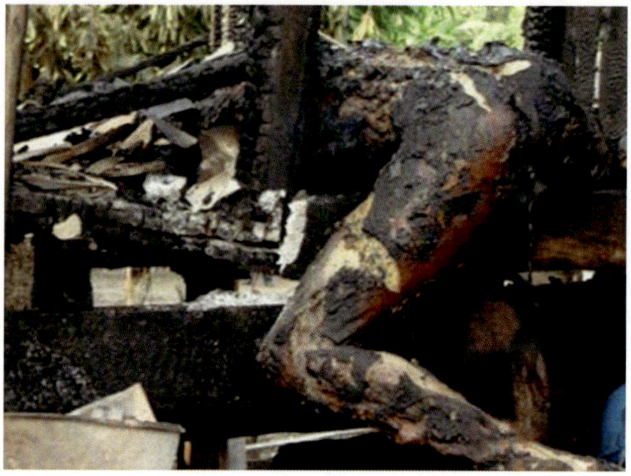

Fig. 3.28

important to note that this should be accomplished only after proper notation of the location of the fragment(s) has been made.

Decomposed Body

The decomposed body generally has the oral structures intact, but the decomposition process in many cases will cause the fibers which hold the teeth to the bone in the dental arches to break down. With this breakdown of the periodontal fibers, the teeth, especially those with straight roots (like the front teeth), can be easily dislodged and potentially lost prior to examination. Before moving the body, note the absence of any front teeth by separating the lips gently. If some are missing from open sockets, look to see if there are any teeth near the body. If not, those teeth may be found later during the examination. They are often located at the back of the mouth. If not found, the sight of the body should be revisited and searched for the missing evidence. Caution must be taken when moving the body so that any loose teeth are not inadvertently bumped and dislodged.

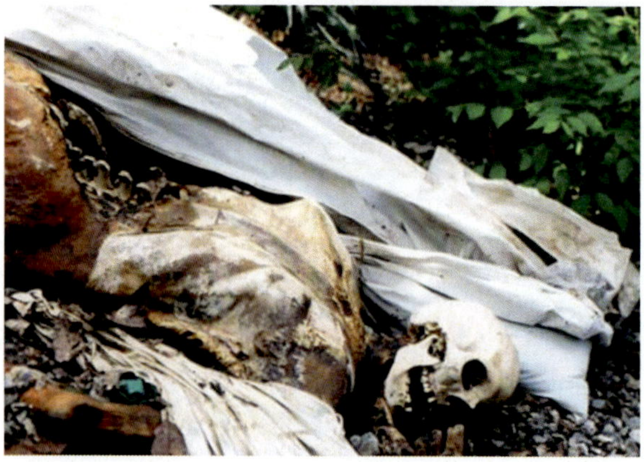

Fig. 3.29

Severely Burned Body

- In all severely burned cases, extreme caution must be taken in transporting the body, not because whole teeth will dislodge but because the heat may have so desiccated and charred the crowns of the teeth that merely touching them may cause them to shatter. If the teeth appear likely to be fragile, close-up photographs of the dentition prior to careful transport may be helpful in reconstruction, if there is damage during the movement of the body.

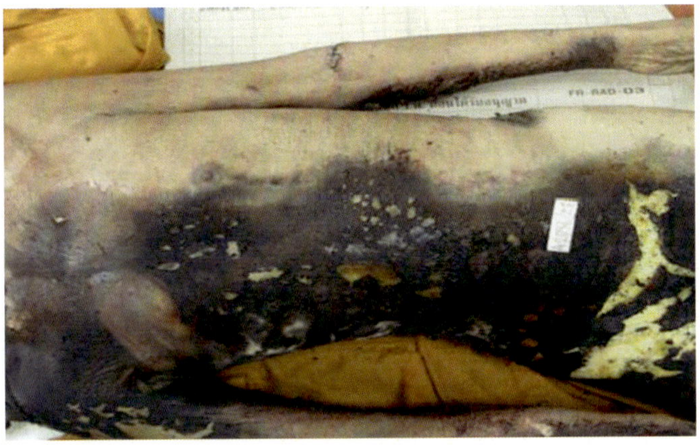

Fig. 3.30

- Above all, great care should be taken not to jar the body during transport. All surrounding debris which might contain dental evidence should be recovered as well, so that it can be inspected for dental fragments. Once in the examination facility, it is sometimes possible to reinforce the dental structures so that they are not as likely to fracture by spraying an adhesive over the teeth. Attempts to maintain as much intact tooth structure and its supporting bone may be critical in verifying the identity of the victim.

Skeletonized Body

In skeletonized cases, the teeth are readily visible but as in the decomposed cases, the soft tissue attachment between the teeth and the bone is no longer holding the teeth in the skeleton. Therefore, straight rooted teeth are easily and often lost. If the body has been buried or animal activity has caused the skeleton to be moved, it may be advisable to shift the surrounding ground for small bones, teeth or other evidence. These fragments can be tagged and brought to the facility for examination.

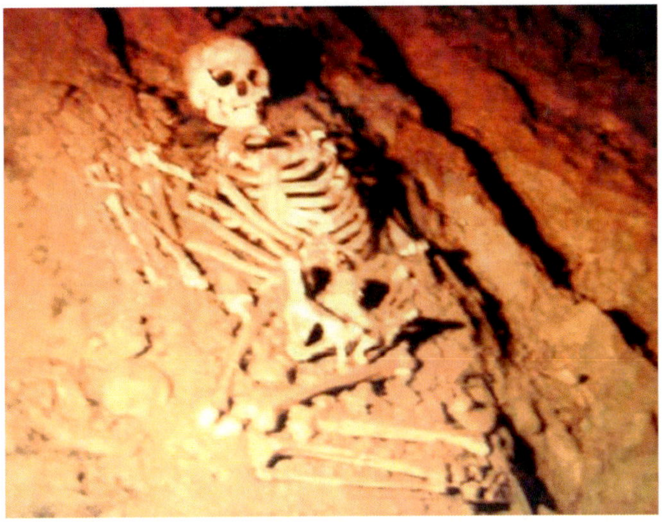

Fig. 3.31

VISUAL EXAMINATION AND DENTAL CHARTING

- This procedure is fairly straight-forward. A complete visual inventory and written record of the remaining dental evidence is basic to any forensic dental examination. The investigating dentist should now record any and all oral and dental features on a form designed for that purpose. This will form the basis for later comparisons in both verification and search activities.

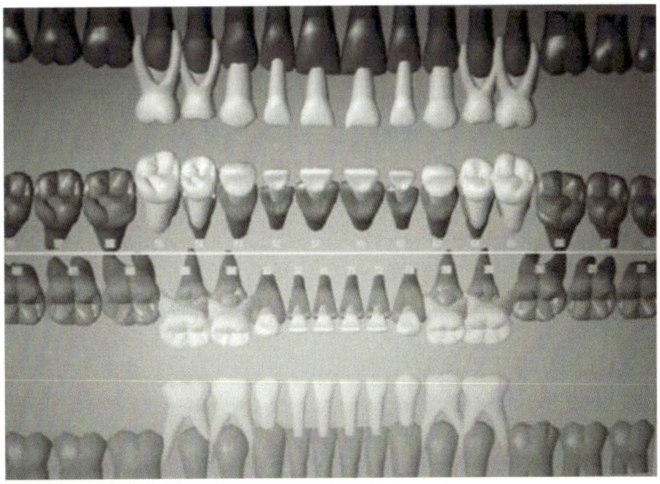

Fig. 3.32

- The actual diagrammatic dental chart used is relatively unimportant. However, whatever chart is employed should allow enough space for adequate notation in either words and/or diagrams of all the existing conditions. It is also recommended that all charting designations for the individual teeth be made in the "universal numbering system."

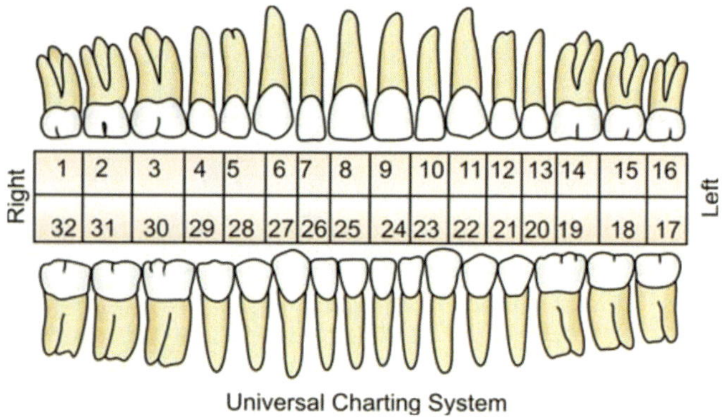

Fig. 3.33

- The visual examination and subsequent dental charting can be a relatively easy procedure or a very tedious, difficult task, depending on the accessibility of the teeth and the condition of the remains. Where all of the teeth remain in the body arches, forcing the jaws open, in some cases breaking the rigor mortis,and cleaning the teeth is all that is necessary. In cases of severe burning, it is sometimes necessary to carefully remove the upper and lower jaws so that cleaning and complete examination may be performed.

Dental Radiographs

- Every postmortem dental examination should include the taking of dental radiographs (X-ray films). The reasons for this are two fold. First, a completely accurate dental charting without radiographs is not possible, since there are many conditions that are only detectable by this method, i.e. root canals, retained roots, impacted teeth, etc. And secondly, dental films are the hard evidence that will be needed to substantiate any conclusions in the case. Anyone can make recording errors on a chart. The radiographs are solid objective recordings of the actual dental characteristics.

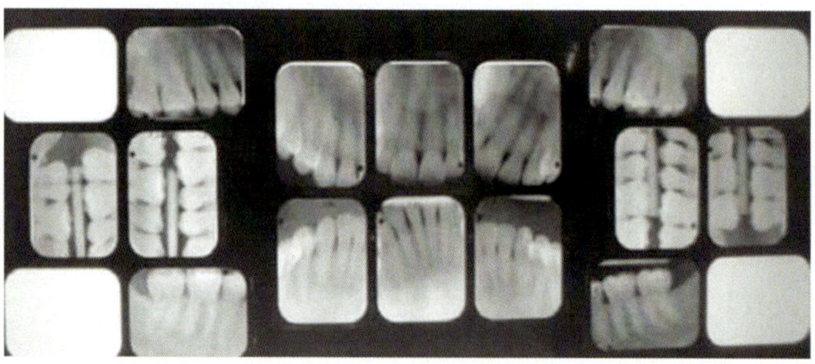

Fig. 3.34

- A thorough postmortem dental radiographic examination should include a complete series of periapical films of the available dental structures. Bitewing type films should also be included since they are the most common type found in dental records. No matter what types are taken, it is important that any films be properly angulated, well-exposed, and well-processed (developed and fixed).
- Besides periapicals and bitewings, there are several other different types of films available. These include panoramics, occlusals, and medical type films, such as lateral head and anterior/posterior skull views.

Bitewing Radiographs

These are the most common type of radiograph found in dentistry and therefore, likely to turn-up as part of the antemortem dental record. In fact, quite often it is the only type of dental film available. Because they are taken of both jaws at the same time (in occlusion), these films generally show the upper and lower teeth in close approximation, therefore depicting the full crowns of all of the teeth visible in the exposure. These films do not show the areas around the ends of the roots and therefore may not disclose some very useful information. If the jaws and teeth are severely fragmented or the teeth are very fragile, it may be difficult to secure radiographs of this type for the postmortem dental record. Nonetheless, every effort should be made to include bitewings in the examination.

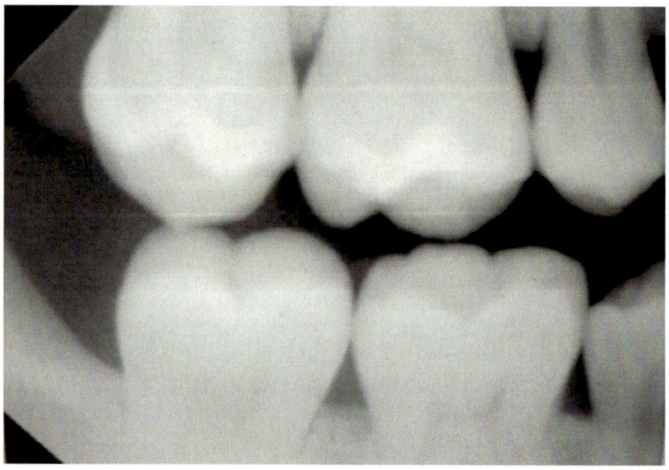

Fig. 3.35

Periapical Radiographs

The periapical dental film is taken of one jaw at a time, and it shows the bony structure at and around the end of the root as well as the entire tooth itself. Depending on the location and condition of the individual, usually two to four teeth will show fairly completely on one of these films. These should be taken in all areas of the dental arches, even those not containing visible teeth, since teeth or other characteristics can be impacted or hidden within the bony structures. A full set of these films should be taken along with any bitewing films. A full set of periapical films will usually include about fourteen films of the standard dental size.

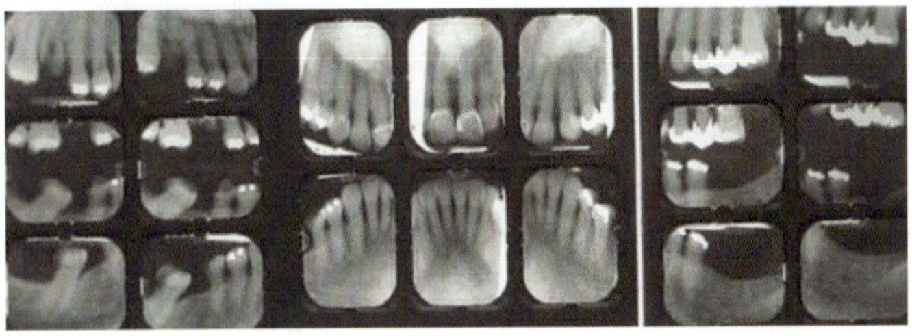

Fig. 3.36

Panoramic Radiographs

This type of film provides a large single radiograph that shows most of the lower face including both jaws, the sinus cavities, nasal passages, lower portions of the eye sockets, and the angles of the mandible. The film is taken with the head stabilized in a cradle while the X-ray source and the film cassette both travel around the head. These films are not routinely taken in most dental offices. However, they are common enough that their use in forensics has to be considered. They should be used for comparison to antemortem dental films cautiously, if the antemortem films are of a different type. This is because: (1) The film is so large that individual teeth and supporting structures are often overlapped and/or distorted, making comparison to other film types difficult; (2) The sheer logistics of positioning a decedent's head, jaw or jaw fragments, onto the machine may prevent the production of a quality image.

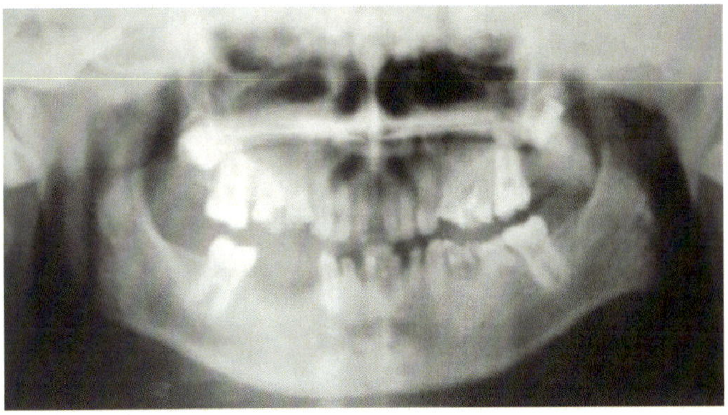

Fig. 3.37

Medical Radiographs

These films are those radiographs commonly taken for orthodontic purposes or for diagnosis of head injuries, sinus problems and the like. These films usually show the entire skull from a particular view or exposure. While anatomical features such as the sinuses, especially the frontal sinus in an anterior/posterior view of a Waters view, can be beautifully depicted, the visualization of the teeth is difficult due to overlapping of teeth, superimposition of the right and left sides of the arches and other types of distortion. All of these factors can make comparison of specific dental features very difficult.

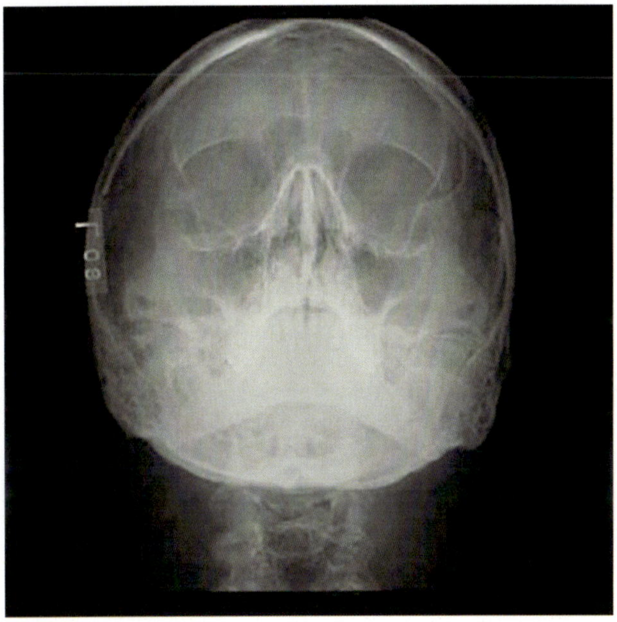

Fig. 3.38

Photographs

Although generally not as critical as the dental radiographs, dental photographs are very helpful in preserving the evidence, especially when there is some unique dental feature which would be difficult to describe otherwise. Photography can also provide a double check for possible recording errors. In addition, photographs, particularly those of the front teeth, may be useful for comparisons to antemortem photographs which show unusual features of these teeth. These photographs should include all those views that the investigating forensic dentist feels are important.

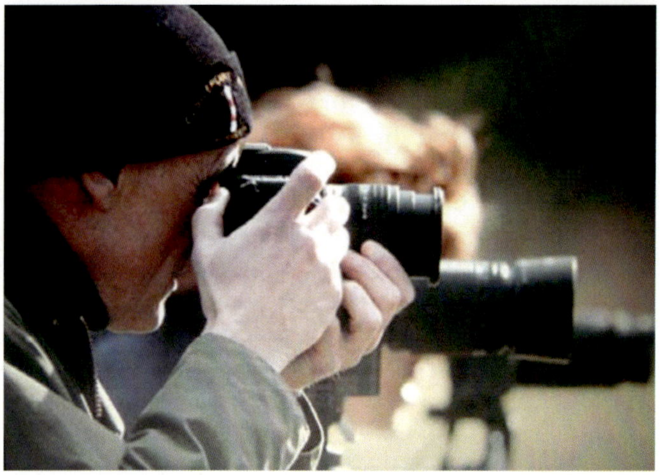

Fig. 3.39

Study Models

Study models are seldom used to preserve evidence in identification cases. Due to fragility of the teeth in some situations and the breakdown of the soft tissue in others, taking impressions can, under certain circumstances, alter the existing evidence. However, for any given particular case, it may be a procedure that the examining forensic dentist would feel is necessary.

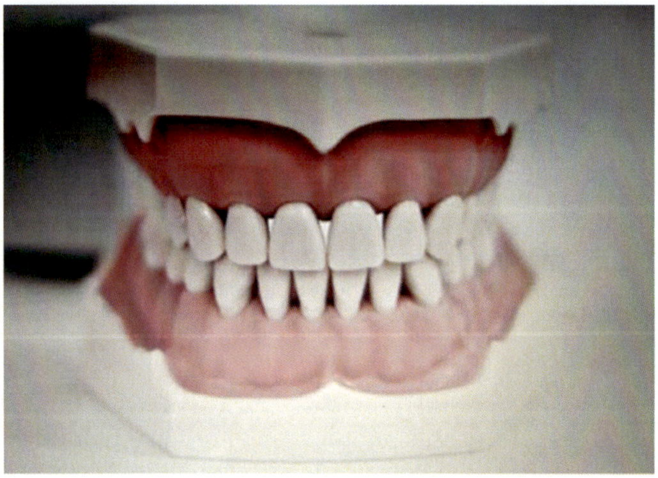

Fig. 3.40

Preservation of Jaw and Tooth Fragments

In those cases where the dental evidence is minimal or questionable in some way, and/or if the body is to be disposed of by cremation, the dental evidence should be removed from the remainder of the body, marked and properly stored for future examination and study.

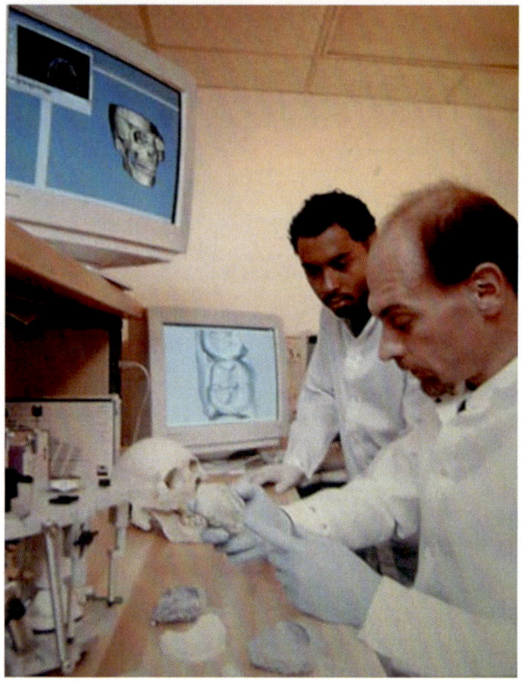

Fig. 3.41

Skeletal Ramains

- These specimens should be thoroughly cleaned and stored in such a way as to insure retention of all dental evidence, keeping in mind that teeth are easily lost from their sockets.
- If necessary resect or remove the jaws from the supporting bone and muscle attachments. The specimen must be cleaned and then stroed in a standard morgue formalin solution.

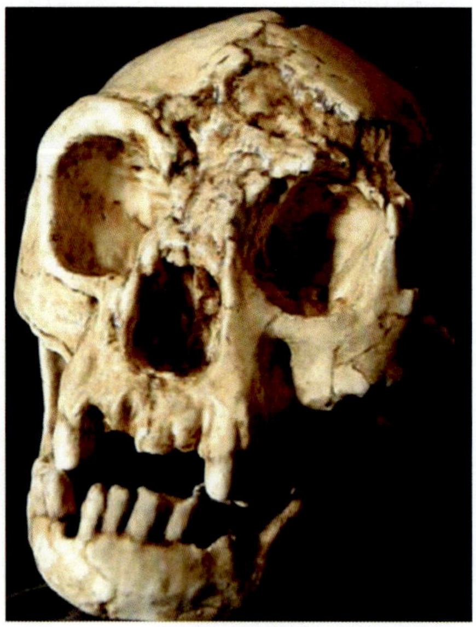

Fig. 3.42

Authorization for Removal of Dental Structures

Resection of the deceased remains will require legal authorization before proceeding. The form of that authority will vary depending on the jurisdiction in which the examination occurs. At the very least it is necessary to obtain permission for the resection from Coroner/Medical Examiner under whose authority the case falls. The methods of resection will vary with the situation and will include use of an autopsy saw, mallet and chisel, or pruning shears. A forensic dentist will be familiar with the technique most applicable to each particular case.

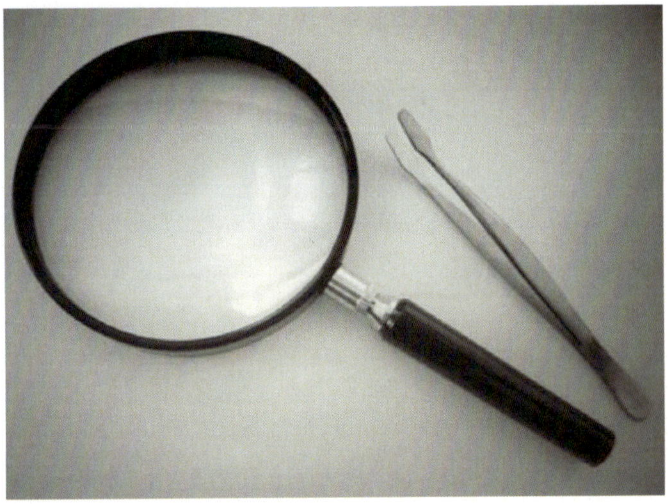

Fig. 3.43

Unidentified Body Report

- Whenever a deceased body is discovered and especially when a timely identification is not anticipated, all available identifying physical evidence needs to be gathered and preserved. This should be accomplished before the body leaves the custody of the responsible investigative authorities. Besides fingerprints, photographs and DNA samples, dental information should be recorded in all cases involving a death, whenever there may be some present or future need to verify the identity of the individual with a degree of scientific certainty.
- Though it is usually the burned, decomposed, or severely traumatized case that ultimately requires dental identification, there is always the possibility that dental verification may be the only scientific method available in other less obvious cases. The Conscientious Investigator should never allow an unidentified body to be disposed of without taking fingerprints, if available. So it should be with any available dental evidence.
- In addition, with the increasing use of computer-based Dental Comparison Programs, it may be that the ultimate clue to the true identity may come from the dental evidence. Rapid identification can be critical in case resolution.
- A trained forensic odontologist should be retained to perform the examination and necessary record-taking, so that all recorded information is accurate, complete and preserved properly. It is always best to do this immediately, and to do it right. This will greatly reduce the necessity of having to exhume the body at a later date and thereby incurring additional expenses, and embarrassment. Be complete and be accurate.

It should be noted here that law enforcement should expect the following from any dental consultant that they employ:

- A written forensic dental report of findings, recommendations and conclusions.
- Copies of all documentation, including charting, photographs, models and radiographs.

Using the Dental Information

Once all of the postmortem records are complete, these should become part of the unidentified persons file in the Coroner/Medical Examiner's Office. The logical next step after the report is completed is to have the consulting forensic dentist compare this newly acquired dental data with any available antemortem information. If no local match is found immediately, the information should be shared with other local, regional, and national agencies which are equipped to handle this type of data.

SEARCH/COMPARISON COMPUTER PROGRAMS

Purpose

- In most cases, the dental identification of unknown human remains is simply a matter of directly comparing the postmortem dental records with the antemortem dental records of a suspected individual. Another more difficult case scenario might involve the discovery of a body when a possible identity is not apparent. In these instances some type of evidence found at the scene or on the body is used.
- One of the most difficult, but more important tasks, that a forensic dentist can be asked to accomplish is the identification of unidentified remains when the investigators have no idea of the possible identity. There are no leads to follow or possible acquaintances to interview. Until the development of computer technologies, this task was all but impossible.

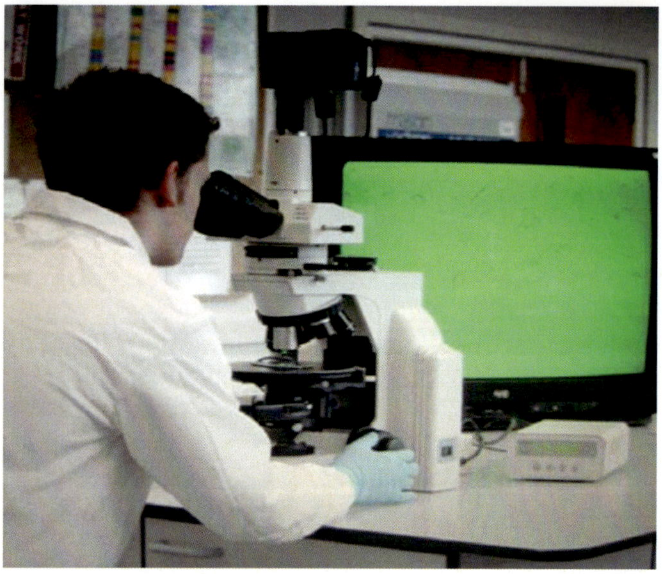

Fig. 3.44

- With the use of computer comparison programs the antemortem and postmortem information can be entered into a data base and thousands of comparisons can be made in seconds generating a list of possible candidates, which can then be confirmed or rejected by visual comparison of the appropriate dental radiographs and/or other dental evidence. For this to be a truly effective tool for law enforcement, appropriate dental search/comparison facilities must exist. Without a useable, up to date data base, the various search procedures can not be accomplished.

Minimum Requirements

- The computer software program must be easy to use and have the capability to perform general and specific searches and dental characteristic comparisons.
- The entry codes, forms, and procedures must be clear and uncomplicated, to reduce data errors.
- Law enforcement offices with authority to submit data must be educated concerning the use and value of the program.
- Mandatory reporting should be required of all law enforcement offices.

CAPMI4 COMPUTER PROGRAM

- Using CAPMI4 (Computer-aided Postmortem Identification) as a parallel system for entry and search of missing and unidentified persons information. This software program was originally developed by the US Army under the direction of Dr Lewis Lorton and programmed by Mr Robert Weed. It was originally developed to assist in mass casualty events and has been used to aid in the identification of remains from the Vietnam and Korean Wars. After ten years of experience using this program, M/UPU has found it to be a very valuable and effective tool in the task of identifying the more difficult cases, where other leads have not been available to investigators.

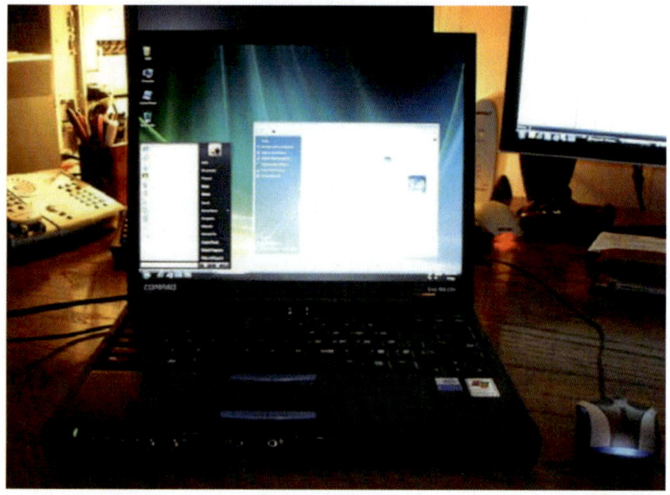

Fig. 3.45

- The choice of CAPMI4 as the tool over other currently available programs is mainly based on its ability to perform accurate search and comparison routines. Supporting this is a long history of development and successful use by CILHI. It has also been used successfully in the identification of missing and unidentified persons in Washington State. The use of a DOS-based computer is also important in that this type of machine is more compatible with machines already in use by Investigating Agencies in the United States and around the world. The program also has design features that allow searches not only for dental characteristics, but also for physical attributes of the individuals, which other programs for dental comparisons may not be capable of accomplishing.

INTER-PROGRAM PROTOCOL

- An issue that has received little attention in the past is the manner in which dental information should be shared between similar search/comparison programs. This has not been addressed because there have been few established programs anywhere. As this changes and as additional facilities come "on line", it will be important to have consistent and practical protocols for sharing of missing and unidentified person information.

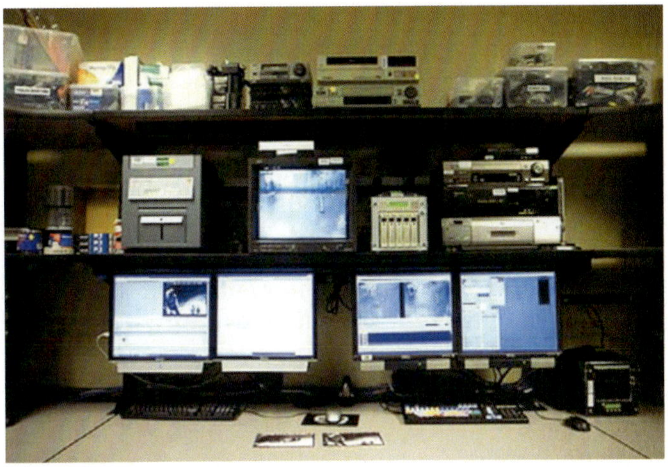

Fig. 3.46

- When developing and implementing interagency protocols a few important factors need to be considered.
- There will always be considerably more missing person cases than unidentified body cases.
- The final verification should only be made and announced by the local jurisdicton and its forensic experts.
- Most, if not all, search/comparison programs will be publicly funded, so successes need to be properly publicized to insure continuance of the programs.

SUGGESTED PROTOCOLS

Sharing Information

- It is important that agencies share the available information with other like programs. Without this type of unselfish exchange of data, no interstate identifications can be accomplished. It is also important to remember that an office that is reluctant to cooperate will soon find cooperation as well. Success is dependent on working together for the good of the public that is being served.
- The questions of which information should be shared with other agencies, and when, is at the heart of the protocol issue.
- The numbers of missing person cases and the volatility of this data base, makes sharing of this information somewhat impractical with all other agencies. However, those programs that have a strong working relationship and reasonable proximity may decide that this exchange will be of some benefit to them.
- Unidentified body case information should be sent to all known agencies with similar programs.
- Once a case has been resolved, all agencies should be similarly advised.
- When Matches Are Discovered:
  - As outlined hare, it is important that the local agency and its forensic expert actually make the final verification of identity. If this is not allowed to occur, it will be a certainty that local office will no longer participate in the program. It is also important that all parties be properly recognized for their participation.
- Suggested protocol when a match is found by a search/comparison program:
  - Notify local agencies.
  - Provide necessary information for verification.
  - Local agency should make final verification and publicize findings, if appropriate.
  - All agencies involved should receive public recognition.

ABFO IDENTIFICATION GUIDELINES

- Collection and Preservation of Postmortem Dental Evidence
  - The remains-examination procedures
  - Photography
  - Jaw resection
  - Techniques for dissection/resection
  - Postmortem dental record
- Sources for Antemortem Data
- Comparison of Antemortem and Postmortem Evidence
- Categories and Terminology for Body Identification
  - The necessity for guidelines and standards in the forensic sciences should be obvious. The American Board of Forensic Odontology (ABFO) adopted Guidelines for Bite Mark Analysis on February 21,1984.
  - Forensic dentistry has provided accurate identifications in mass disasters and in routine cases over the past years, but there have been cases where misidentification have occurred. The objective of these guidelines is to provide guidance to the forensic dentist and are dedicated to the concept of greater accuracy in forensic dentistry.
  - The Body Identification Guidelines have received general acceptance by diplomates of the ABFO, following a preliminary draft by the committee. It is not the purpose of these guidelines to invalidate other methods, but rather to describe methods that a majority of investigators employ.

Collection and Preservation

Postmortem Dental Evidence

The postmortem dental examination is conducted by the authority and under the direction of the Coroner/Medical Examiner or his disignee, typically a forensic pathologist.

Thus, the protocol for the collection of postmortem dental evidence, particularly decisions to incise the facial tissues for access or resect the jaws, is subject to approval by the regional Coroner/Medical Examiner. The actual procedures to be followed in a dental identification case depend in large part on the condition of the remains (as well as other circumstances of the case).

Examination Procedures

- Visually identifiable body
- Photographs
- Radiographs
- Dental charting
- Dental impressions, as applicable
- Resection by inframandibular dissection.
- Decomposed/incinerated body
- Resection and preservation of jaw specimens, if indicated.
- Skeletonized remains.

Photography

Photographic documentation of dental evidence can provide objective data which is often more graphic than the written chart. Photographs (with an accompanying scale) should be taken before and after appropriate cleansing. The ABFO right angle ruler is recommended. The photographs should be clearly labeled with the case number/name and date. All relevant photographic information should be documented.

Recommended Equipment

- Single lens reflex 35 mm camera (The Lester Dine instant close-up camera, model IV, has been useful in mass disaster evidence documentation). Below system and/or lenses for close-up photography. Electronic flash (preferably point flash or ring light system).
- Cheek retractors.
- Intraoral front-surface mirrors.

Film

- Color film (slide and/or print format)
- Black and white film, as required
- Polaroid film may be of help in special circumstances.

Views

- Full face, lips retracted
- Close-up view of anterior teeth
- Lateral views of teeth in slightly open position, and in occlusion
- Occulusal views, upper and lower teeth
- Special views, as required.

Jaw Resection

Facial dissection and/or jaw resection, which may be necessary for full access to dental structures, is done only with approval of the coroner/medical examiner. Circumstances dictating decisions to resect are applicable as follows:

Viewable Bodies

Restricted opening due to rigor may require:

- Intraoral incision of masticatory muscles, with or without fracture of the condyles.
- Breaking the rigor with bilateral leverage on the jaws in the retromolar regions.
- Waiting until the rigor subsides
- Inframandibular dissection with or without mandibular resection.
- Removal of the larynx and tongue at autopsy may facilitate the visual examination of the teeth and placement of intraoral films. Again, the removal of these tissues should only be performed after the autopsy and with permission of the pathologist. These tissues should either be retained by the pathologist or replaced with in the body.

Decomposed, Incinerated, or Fragmented Bodies

Jaw resection in such cases facilitates dental charting and radiographic examination. Careful dissection of the incinerated head, in particular, is required to preserve fragile tooth structure and jaws *in situ*. Radiographs should be made prior to manipulation of badly burned fragments (mechanical or chemical), stabilization of such tissue should be instituted where necessary.

Skeletonized Remains

Once the skull and mandible are readily separated from the remainder of the skeleton, resection of the maxilla is not required.

Preservation of Evidence

- Jaw resection may be indicated in cases in which. Body parts are to be transferred, with proper authorization, to other facilities for additional examination and testing.
- A homicide victim is to be cremated.

Techniques for Dissection/Resection

Selected techniques are described below. Other methods may be employed when indicated.

Facial Dissection

Bilateral incisions of the face. Beginning at the oral commissures and extending posteriorly to the anterior ramus, permit reflection of the soft tissues for better access.

Inframandibular Approach

Bilateral incisions are made across the upper anterior neck and extend to points posterior and inferior to the ears. The skin and underlying tissues are then reflected upward over the lower face thereby exposing the mandible.

JAW RESECTION

Stryker Autopsy Say Method

The soft tissue and muscle attachments on the lateral aspect of the mandible are dissected away by incisions which extend through the mucobuccal fold to the lower border of the mandible. Lingual attachments are similarly incised to include the internal pterygoid attachments to medial aspect of the rami and the masseter attachments on the lateral aspect. On the maxilla, facial attachments are incised high on the malar processes and superior to the anterior nasal spine. Stryker saw cuts are made high on the rami to avoid possible impacted third molars. Alternatively, the mandible may also be removed by disarticulation at the temporomandibular joints. Bony cuts on the maxilla are made high on the malar processes and above the anterior nasal spine to avoid the apices of the maxillary teeth. A surgical mallet and chisel inserted in the Stryker saw cuts in the malar processes and above the anterior nasal spine are used to complete the separation of the maxilla. Remaining soft tissues in the soft palate and fauces are then dissected free.

Mallet and Chisel Method

A mallet and chisel can be used to induce a "Le Fort" Type I fracture of the maxilla. The chisel blows are made below the zygomatic arch, high on the maxillary sinus walls bilaterally. Since it is virtually impossible to fracture the mandibular rami with the mallet and chisel, the mandible can be disarticulated at the temporomandibular joint in such cases.

Pruning Shears Method

An alternative technique for resection of the jaws involves the use of large pruning shears. The small blade of the pruning shears is placed within the nares and forced back into the maxillary sinus. A cut is then made along a plane superior to the apices of the maxillary teeth bilaterally. The mandibular bone cuts are performed by inserting the small blade of the shears high on the lingual aspect of the ramus near the coronoid notch bilaterally.

Postmortem Dental Record

While most morgues will have the standard autopsy equipment, the forensic odontologist may wish to assemble his own forensic kit to include mouth mirrors, explorers, camera equipment, anatomic dental charts, impression materials, etc. Postmortem dental examinations might utilize anatomic dental charts, photographs, radiographs, models, tape recordings and/or narrative descriptions. The data collected should be comprehensive in scope since antemortem records are commonly not discrovered until days, weeks or even years later. Accordingly, the postmortem dental record will include all or most of the items listed.

- Basic data
- Case number
- Date/Time
- Jurisdiction/authority
- Location
- Tentative ID, if any
- Body description, general
- Approximate age
- Race
- Sex
- Condition
- Jaw fragment(s)
- Description
- Dental examination
- The universal conditions, calculus, stain
- Occlusal relationships, malposed teeth; anomalous, congenitally missing and supernumerary teeth
- Intraoral photographs should be used to show anatomic details of teeth restorations, periodontium, occlusion, lesions, etc.

NARRATIVE DESCRIPTION AND NOMENCLATURE

The anatomic dental chart may be supplemented by a narrative description of the postmortem findings with particular emphasis on unusual or unique conditions. Standardized dental nomenclature should be used as follows:

Universal Numbering System

The system of numbering teeth used in the United States. The teeth are numbered from 1 to 32. The upper right third molar is #1, the upper central incisors are #8 and #9, the upper left third molar #16, the lower left third molar #17 and the lower right third molar is #32. The universal tooth numbering system plus the actual name of the tooth should be used (e.g. tooth #3, upper right first permanent molar).

Dentition Type and Tooth Surfaces

- Primary, permanent and mixed dentition.
- Mesial, occlusal, distal, facial and lingual surfaces.
- Prosthetics and other appliances.
- Crowns: Full, 3/4 or 7/8 coverage restorations. Prostheses: Partial, full, or fixed.
- Orthodontic bands, brackets, space maintainers and retainers.
- Mouthguards and nightguards.

The FDI Numbering System

Odontologists should be aware of the FDI system of numbering teeth. This system is used through out the developed world. Quadrants are numbered from 1 to 4. The upper right quadrant is 1, upper left 2, lower left 3 and lower right 4. Teeth are numbered from the midline to the posterior. Central incisors are #1, canines #3 and third molars #8. Teeth are represented by a two digit code with the quadrant first and the tooth second. Thus, the upper left first molar is #26.

Dental Impression

Impressions should be considered when bitemarks, rugae patterns or other evidence warrant the procedure.

Supplies and Equipment

- Appropriate trays, plastic or metal, which can be modified to fit the mouth.
- Alginate or other American Dental Association approved dental impression material.
- Dental stone is the material of choice for pouring models. Plaster of Paris should not be used.

Impressions and Preparation of Models

- Two sets of impressions, both maxillary and mandibular, are obtained in the conventional manner.
- Models should be trimmed and appropriately labeled with the case number and date.

Dental Radiology

Postmortem radiographs graphically complement the visual examination/charting of the oral and perioral structures and can provide significant data essential for identification. In general, radiographs are required in cases where there is no putative ID, antemortem records have not yet been located and/or the jaws can not be retained. Postmortem radiographs must be considered the prime method of identification. A comprehensive postmortem radiographic examination might include all or some of the following views, depending on the circumstances of the case.

Intraoral Radiographs

Bitewing and periapical ragiographs of anterior and posterior teeth comparable to those taken antemortem. (Bitewing views need not be taken in the conventional manner with the teeth in occlusion; rather, periapical film can be used for separate views of the upper and lower teeth, using a horizontal bitewing angulation).

Dental Fragments, Dissociated Teeth

Appropriate radiographs of all dental fragments, dissociated teeth, bone and restorations should be obtained. Occlusal or lateral plate film may be used for objects larger than a periapical film.

Edentulous Areas

- Periapical radiographs of edentulous arches or areas, especially the third molars, which may be impacted or previously extracted.
- Periapical radiographs of sockets of teeth lost postmortem should be taken, since antemortem radiographs of these same teeth may be the only evidence that becomes available.

Extraoral Radiographs

Extraoral radiographs (e.g. lateral jaw, maxillary or frontal sinus and panoramic radiographs) are often useful.

Disposition of radiographs

- Double pack intraoral film is recommended.
- One set of films should be retained by the forensic odontologist for his case file. The second set may be mounted and forwarded with a written report to the Medical Examiner/Coroner for the master file.

Note: All duplicate films should bear right and left notations.

SOURCES OF ANTEMORTEM DATA

- Antemortem data may include as dental radiographs, written records, models and photographs. Original radiographs should be obtained if possible. The discovery and collection of antemortem records is ordinarily the responsibility of the investigative agency who has access to missing persons reports at the local, state or national level. However, the forensic odontologist may recognize additional characteristics (e.g. prior orthodontic treatment) which could be helpful in establishing a potential ID. This section lists a variety of resource agencies and/or individuals that might provide assistance in locating records.
- *Local agencies*
  - Hospitals, other health care facilities.
  - Dental hospitals.
  - Health care providers.
  - Employer dental insurance carrier.
- *State agencies*
  Contact state of local agencies for dental record assistance.
- *Federal agencies*
  - FBI National Crime Information Center (NCIC)
  - Insurance Carriers
  - Other sources
  - Family/friends/coworkers.
  - Public Aid Insurance Administrator.
  - Employer Dental Insurance Carrier.
  - Prior Military Service.
  - Prior Judicial detention in country.
  - State or Federal Institutions
  - Prior Hospitalizations (e.g. chest films, skull films).
  - Oral surgeons in the area.
  - Veterans administration hospitals.
  - Any previous areas of residence.
  - Chiropractice X-rays.
  - If evidence of orthotreatment, orthodontists in the area.
  - Comparison of antemortem and postmortem data.
- This section deals with factors which may be present in both the antemortem and postmortem dental evidence and can be useful for comparison purposes. Most dental identifications are based on restorations, caries, missing teeth and/or prosthetic devices which may be readily documented in the records. It should be noted, however, that the precipitous decrease in caries incidence in recent years will dictate greater reliance on other dental findings in the future. It is emphasized that, given adequate records, a nearly infinite number of objective factor have identification value. Thus, objective findings, particularly those which are unique to the individual, provide the basis for concordance or exclusion.
- Apparent discrepancies between the antemortem and postmortem evidence (e.g. errors in recording dental treatment subsequent to the available antemortem record) must be resolved.
- The following subsections provide examples of objective findings in the teeth, periodontium, and/or jaws, which may be demonstrable in both antemortem and postmortem records. While the factors listed are by no means comprehensive, they may serve as a checklist and demonstrate the range of objective findings that may be applicable in difficult identification cases.

DENTAL FEATURES USEFUL IN IDENTIFICATION

Teeth

- Teeth present

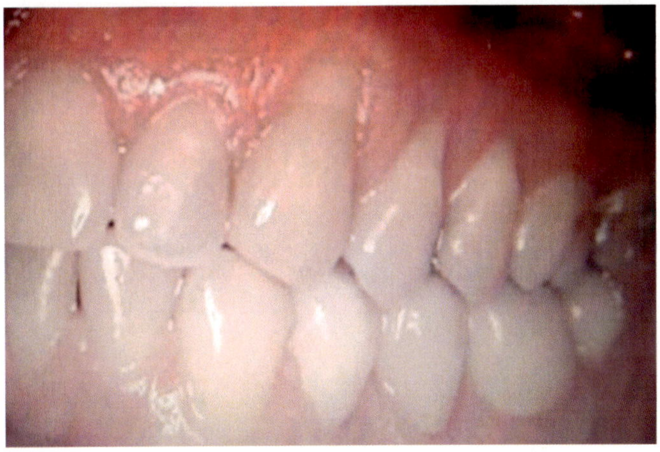

Fig. 3.47

- Erupted

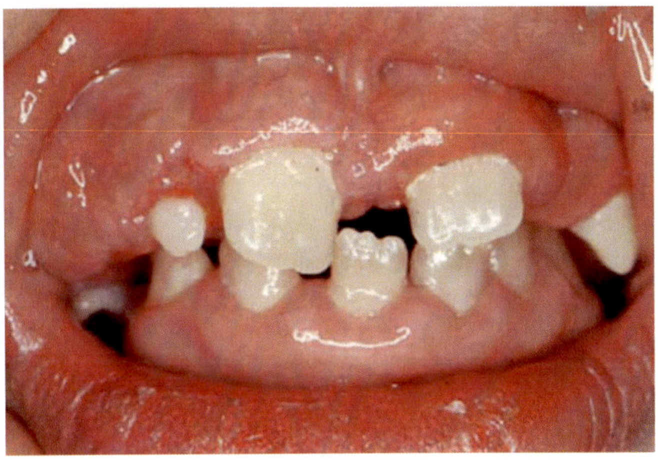

Fig. 3.48

- Unerupted/impacted

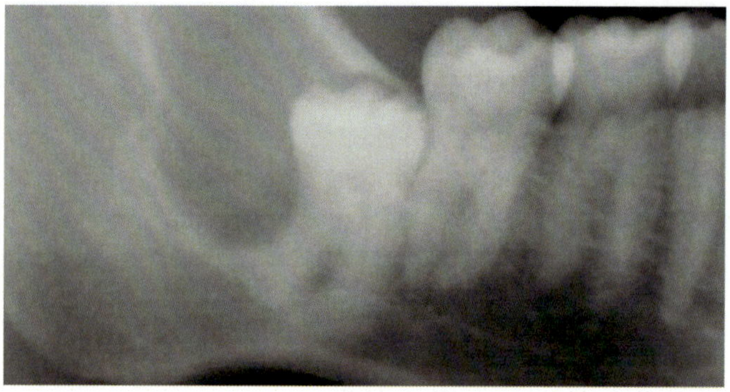

Fig. 3.49

- Missing teeth

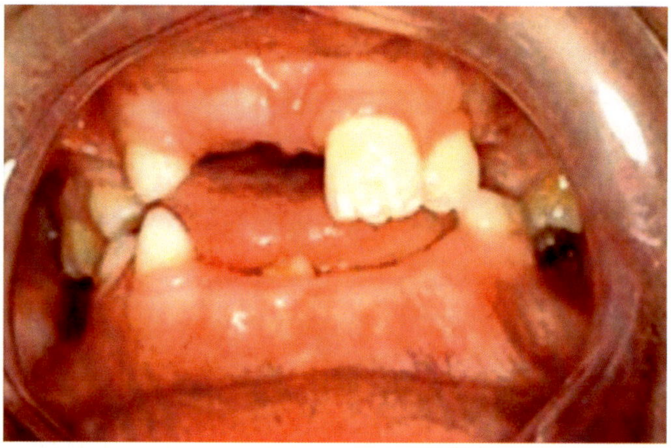

Fig. 3.50

- Congenitally missing

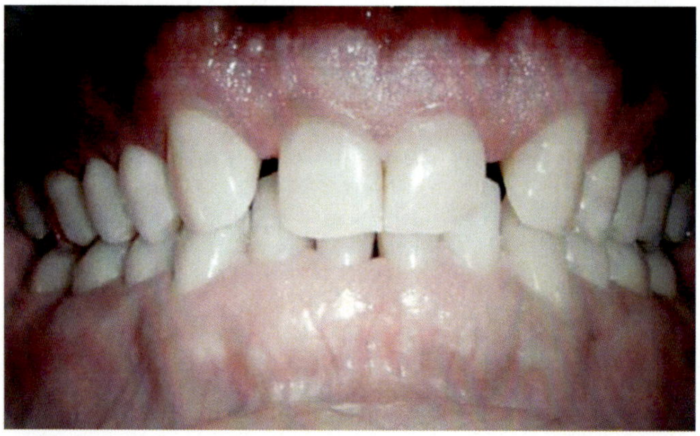

Fig. 3.51

- Tooth Type

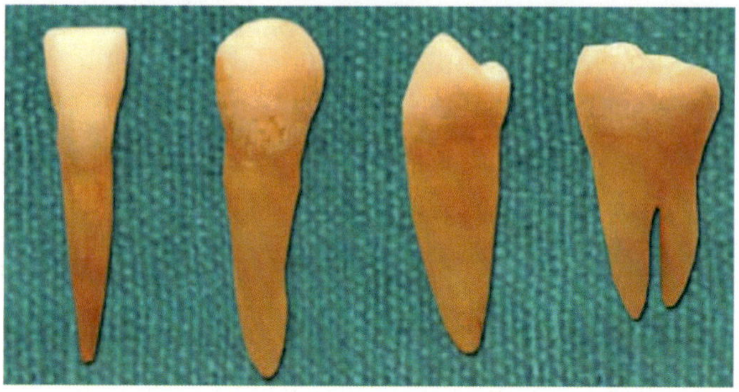

Fig. 3.52

- Permanent

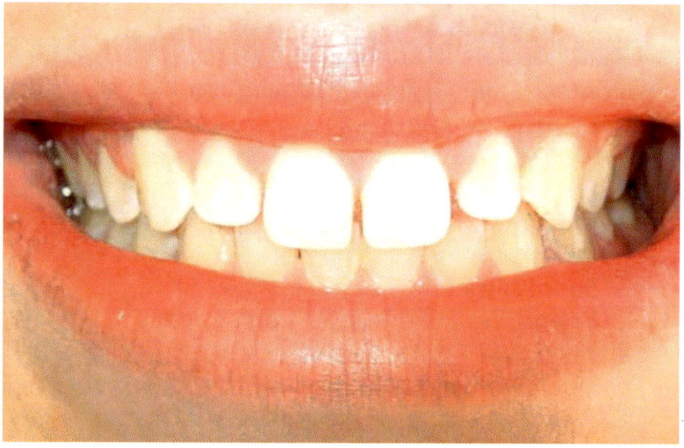

Fig. 3.53

- Mixed dentition

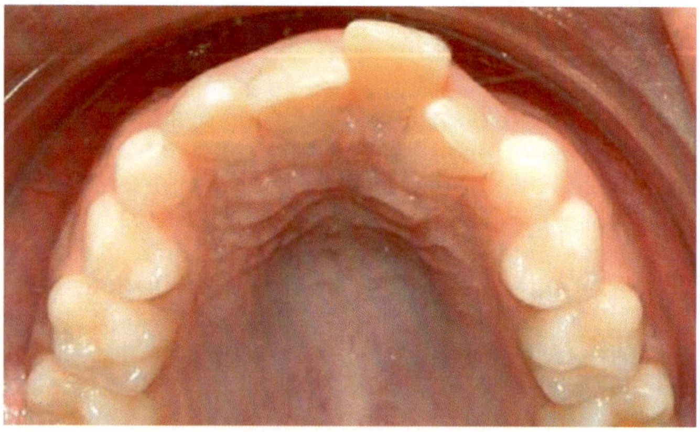

Fig. 3.54

- Retained primary teeth

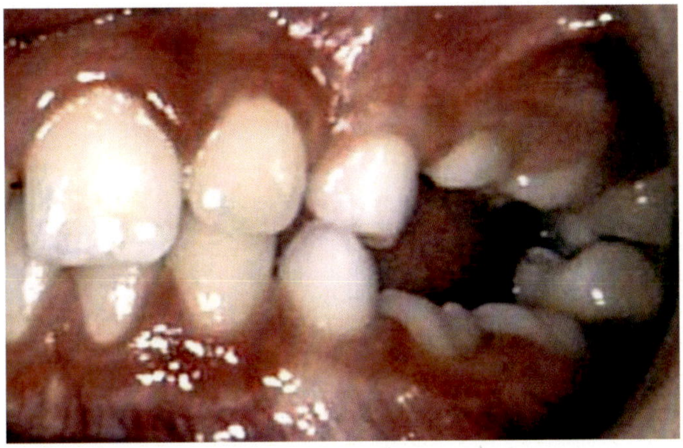

Fig. 3.55

- Supernumerary teeth

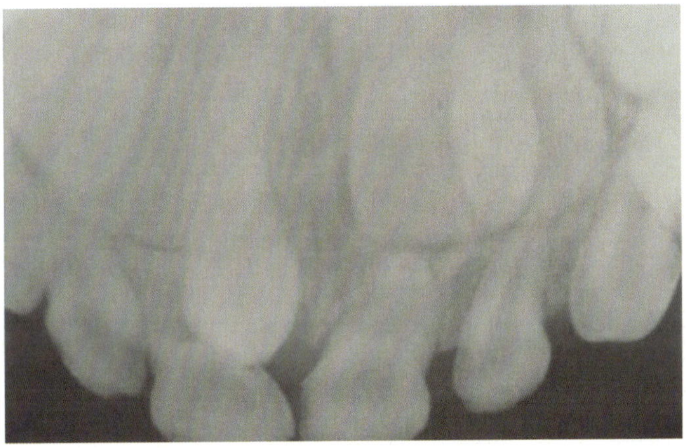

Fig. 3.56

- Tooth Position

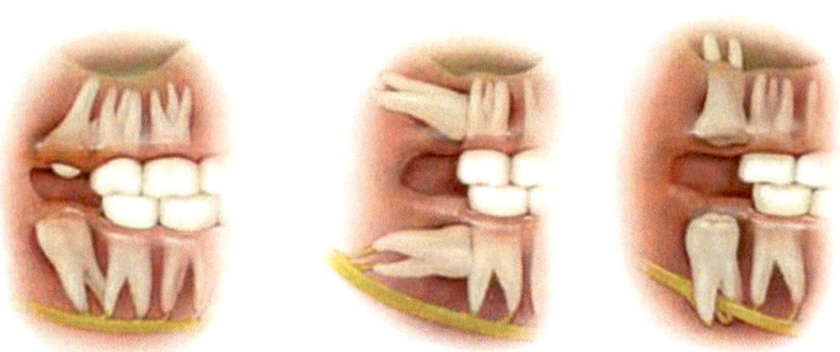

Fig. 3.57

Malpositions

Facial/linguoversion, rotations, supra/infra positions, diastemas, other occlusal discrepancies.

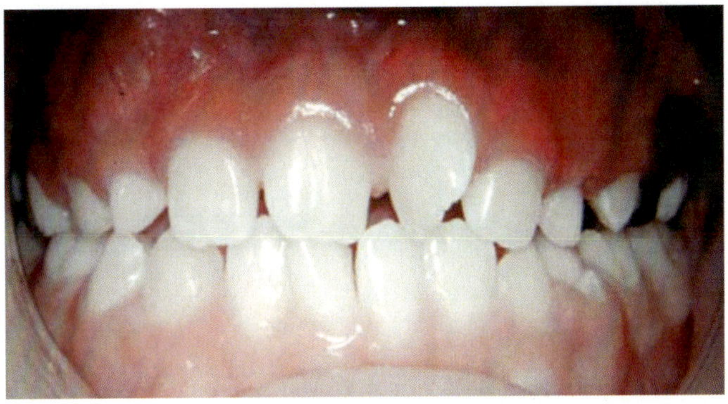

Fig. 3.58

- Crown morphology

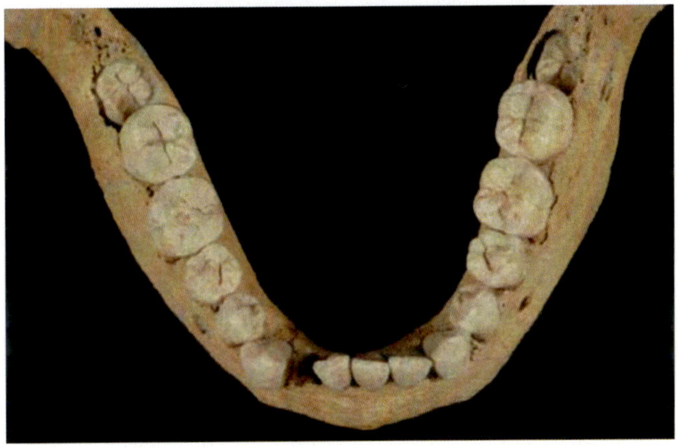

Fig. 3.59

- Size and shape of crowns

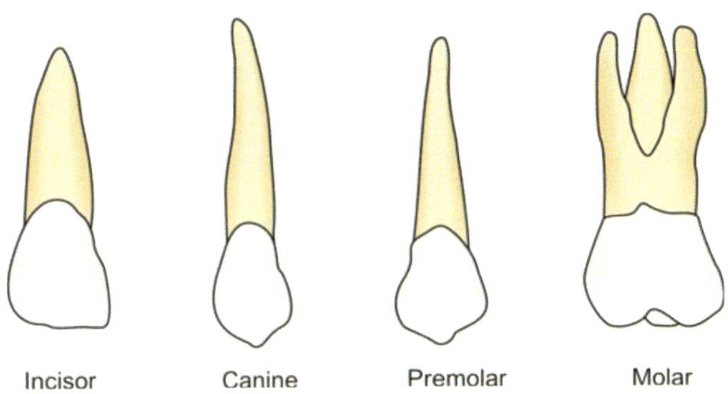

Fig. 3.60

- Enamel thickness, location of contact points, cementoenamel junction.

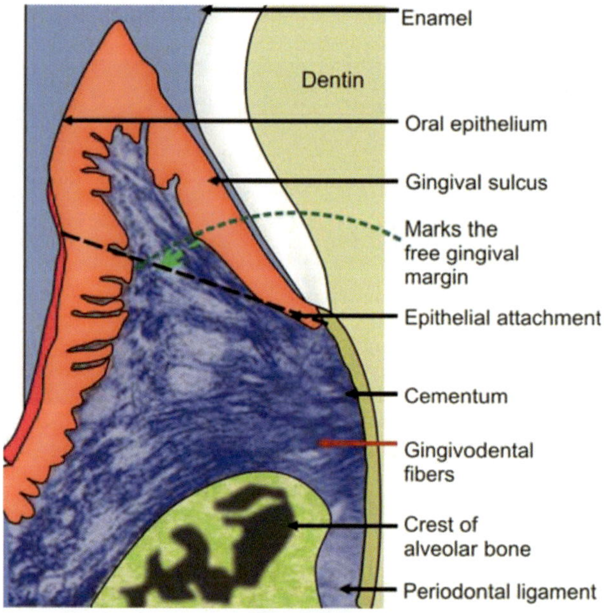

Fig. 3.61

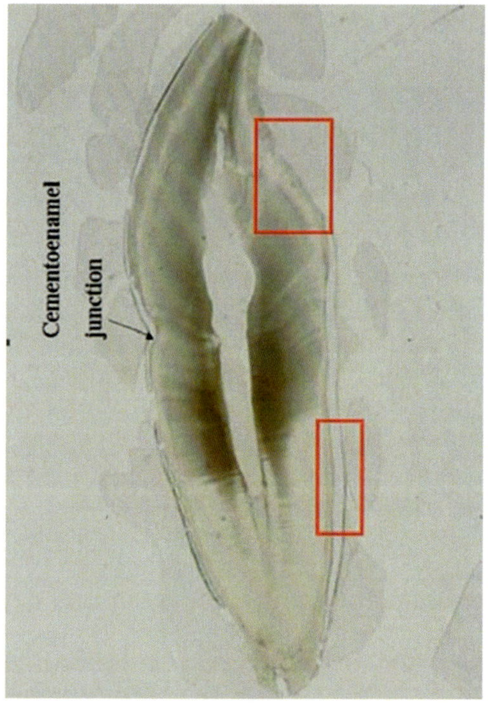

Fig. 3.63

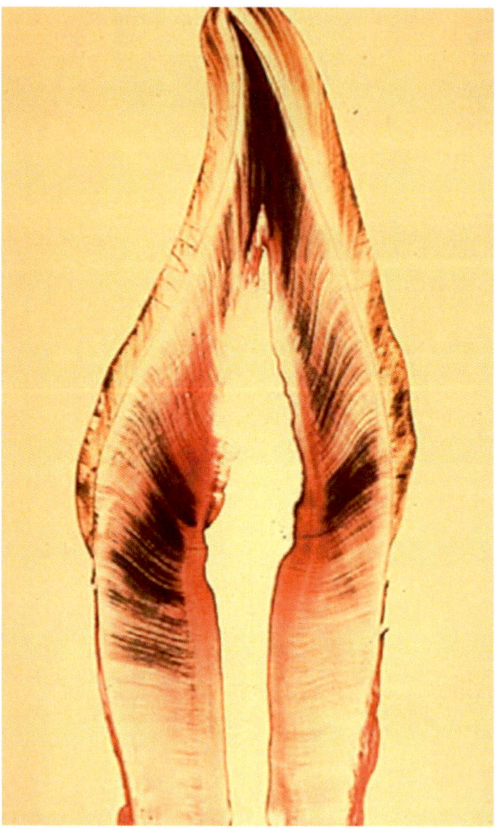

Fig. 3.62

Racial Variations

- Peg laterals

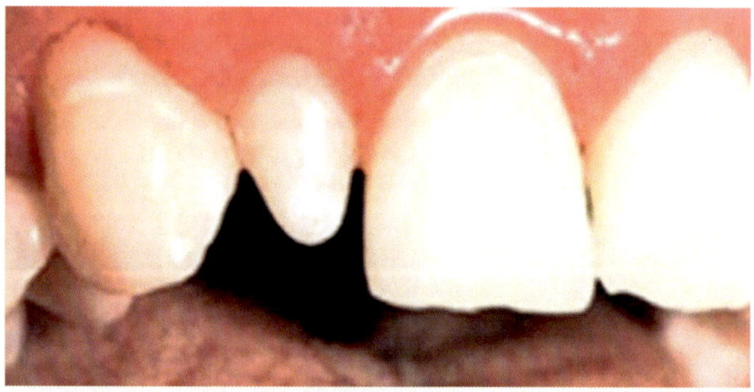

Fig. 3.64

- Fusion/gemination

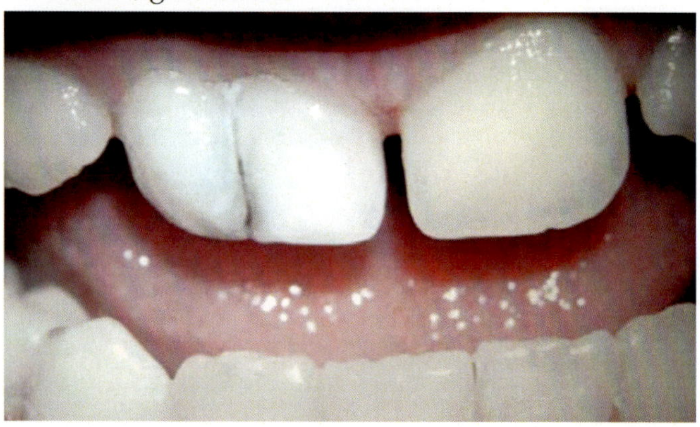

Fig. 3.65

- Enamel pearl

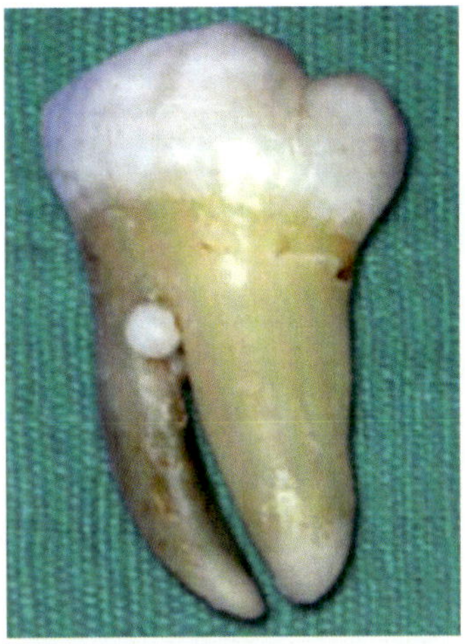

Fig. 3.66

- Dens-in-dente

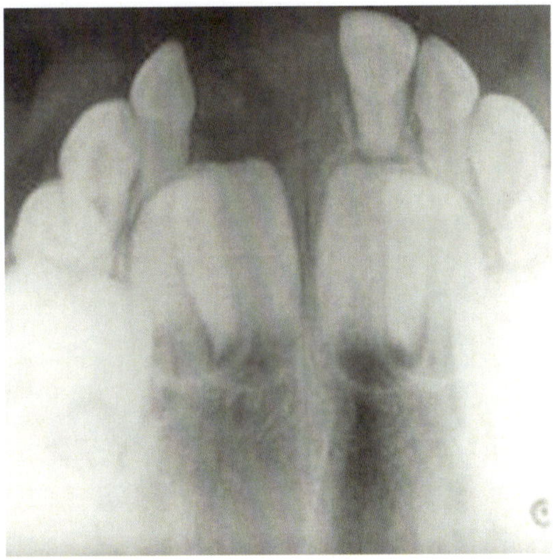

Fig. 3.67

- Dentigerous cyst

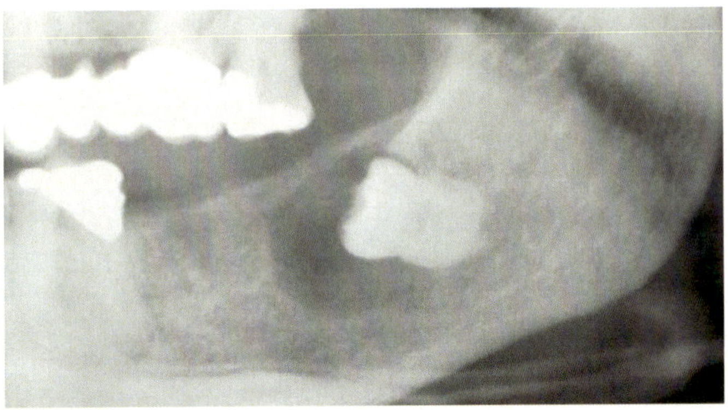

Fig. 3.68

- Root morphology

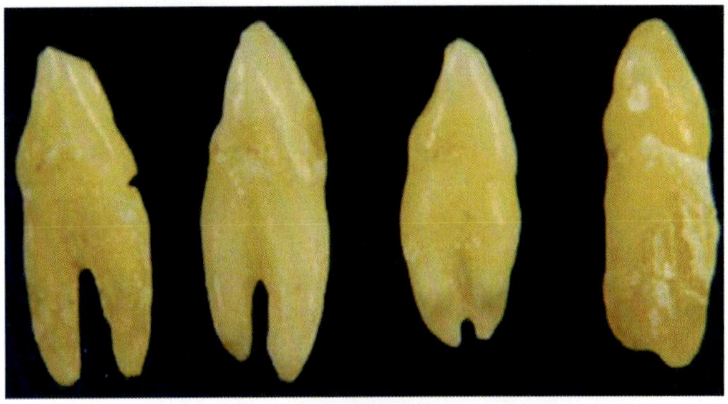

Fig. 3.69

- Size, shape, number, dilaceration, divergence of roots

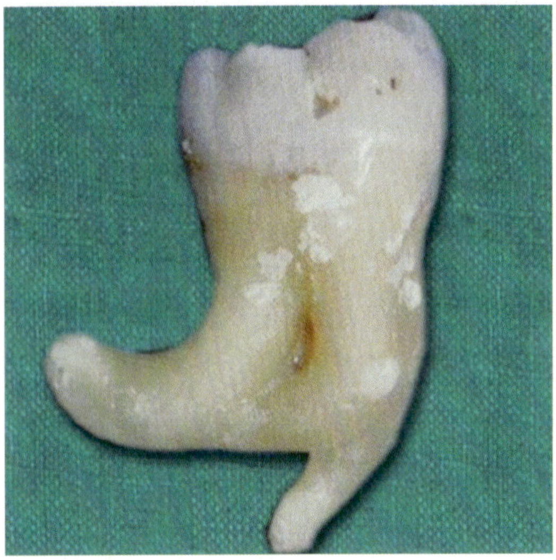

Fig. 3.70

- Root pathology

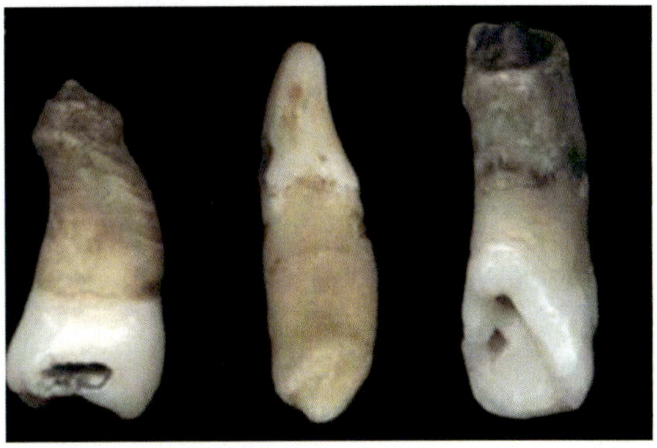

Fig. 3.71

- Root fracture

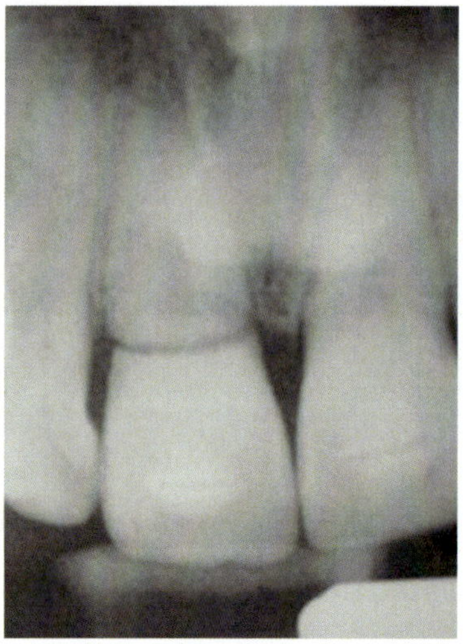

Fig. 3.72

- Hypercementosis

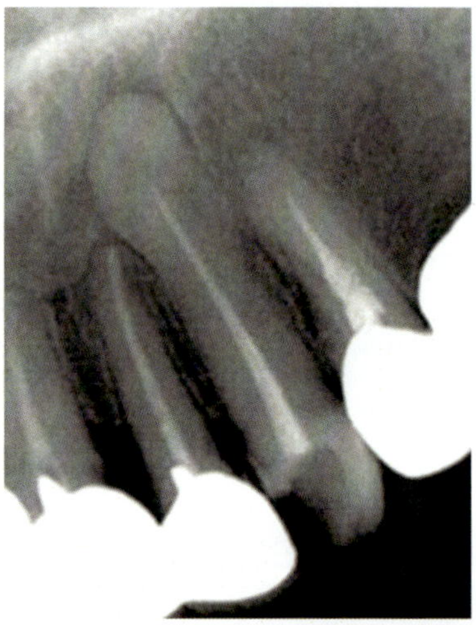

Fig. 3.73

- External root resorption

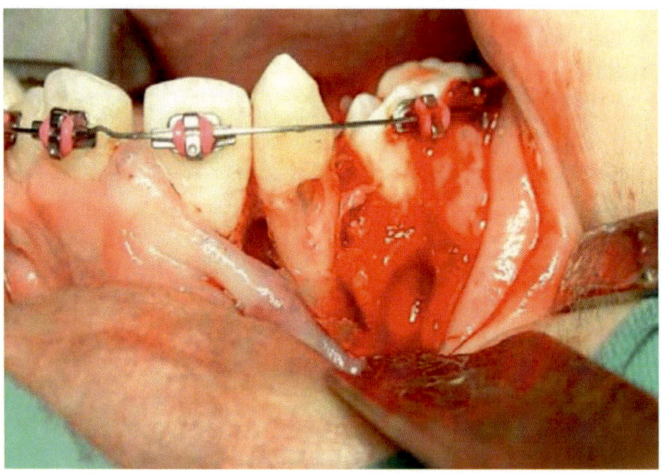

Fig. 3.74

- Root hemisections

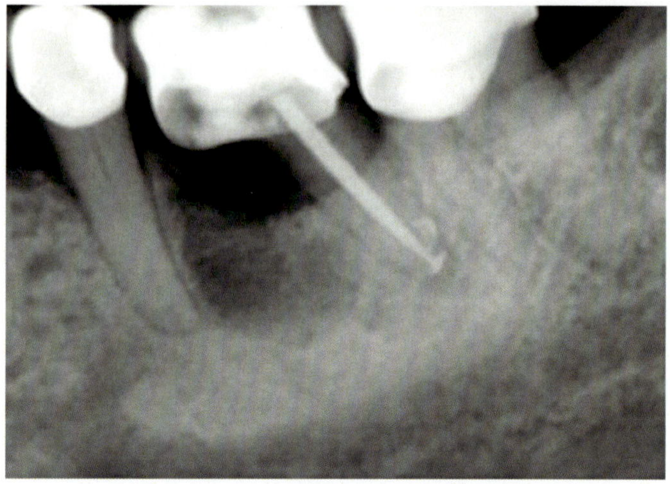

Fig. 3.75

- Pulp chamber and root canal morphology

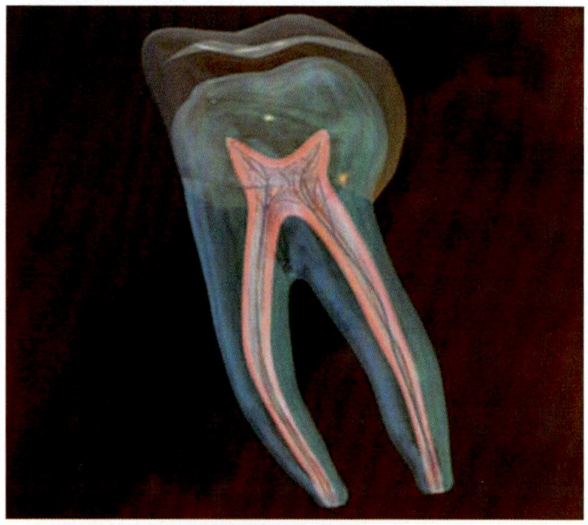

Fig. 3.76

- Size, shape, number

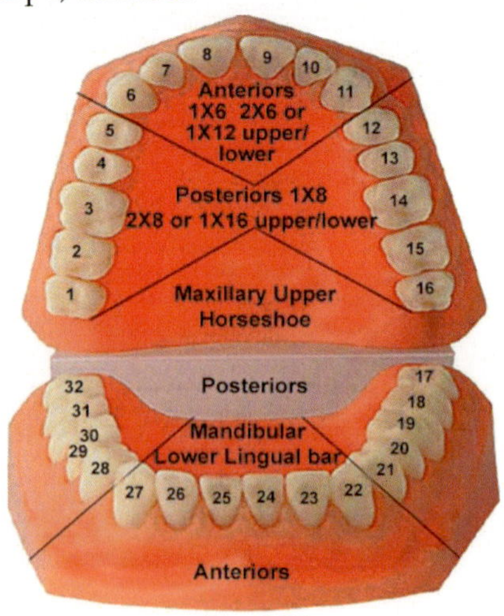

Fig. 3.77

- Secondary dentin

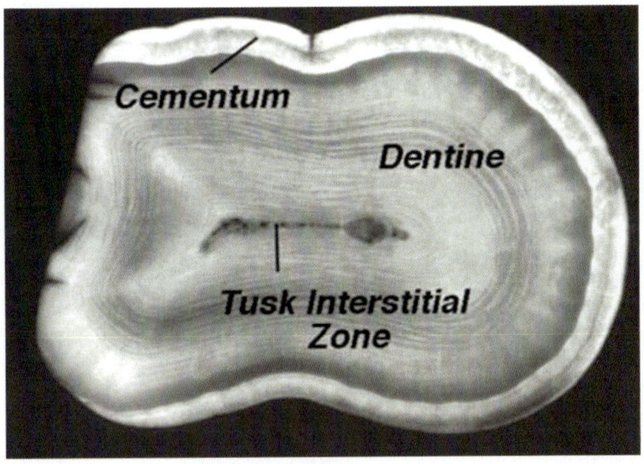

Fig. 3.78

- Pulp stones, dystrophic calcification

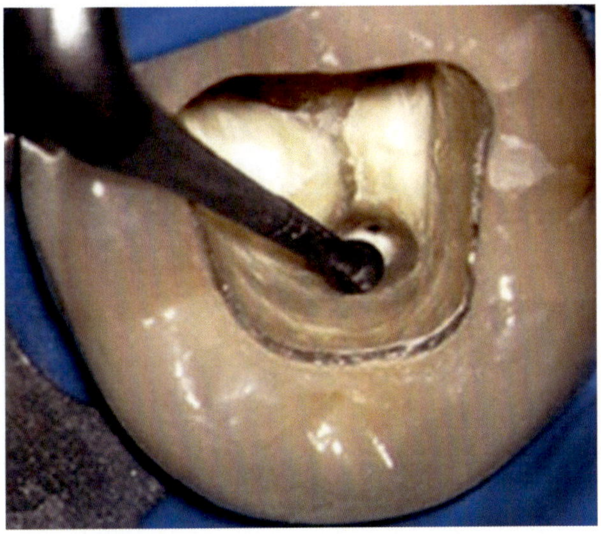

Fig. 3.79

- Root canal therapy: Gutta-percha

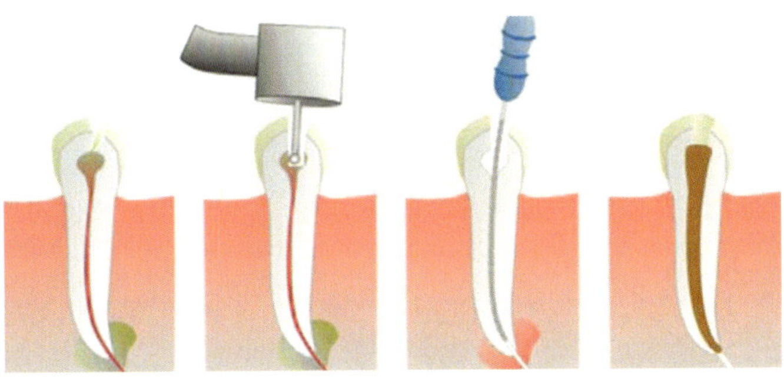

Fig. 3.80

- Silver points, endopaste and retrofill procedures

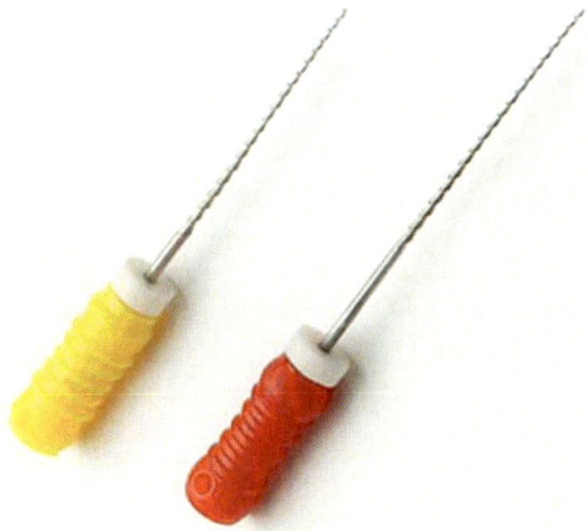

Fig. 3.81

- Internal resorption

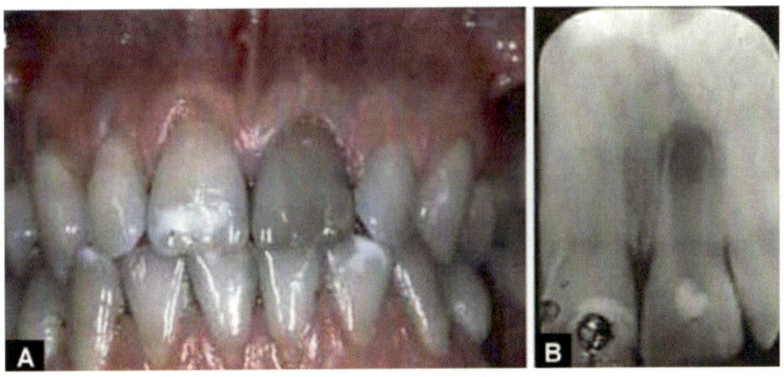

Figs 3.82A and B

- Periapical pathology

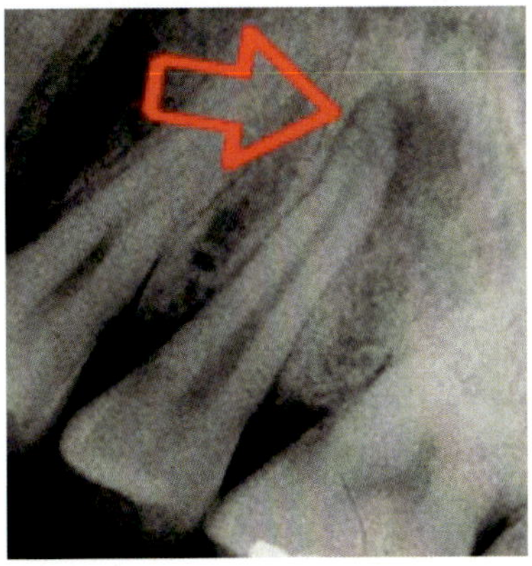

Fig. 3.83

- Periapical abscess/granuloma/cyst

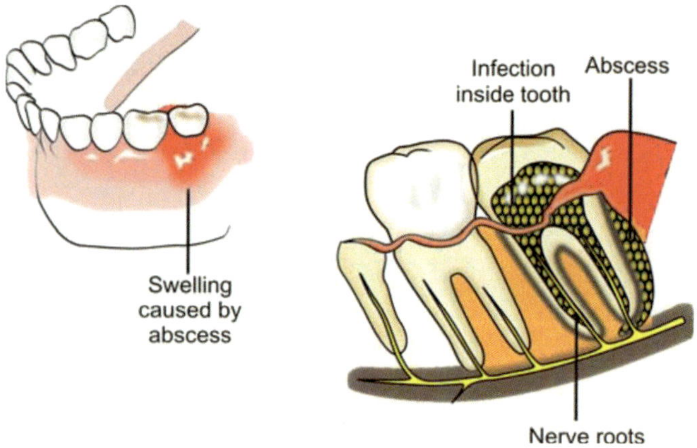

Fig. 3.84

- Cementoma

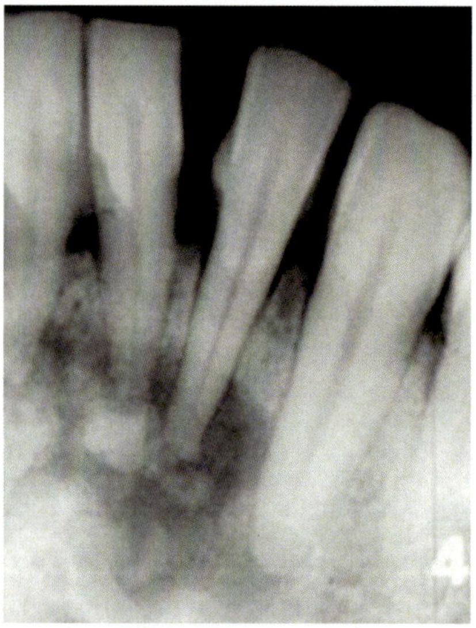

Fig. 3.85

- Condensing osteitis

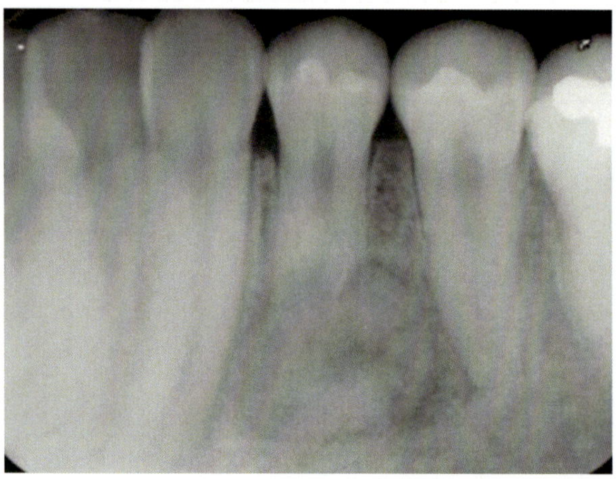

Fig. 3.86

Dental Restorations

- *Metallic restorations:* Amalgams, gold or nonprecious metal crowns/inlays, endoposts, pins, fixed prostheses, implants.

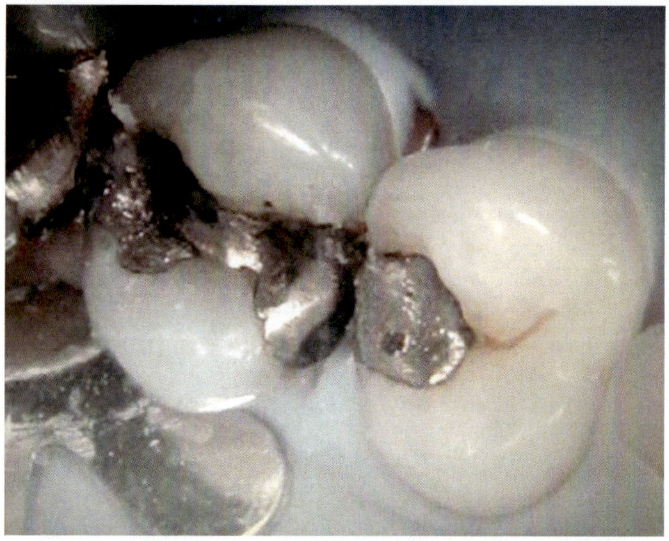

Fig. 3.87

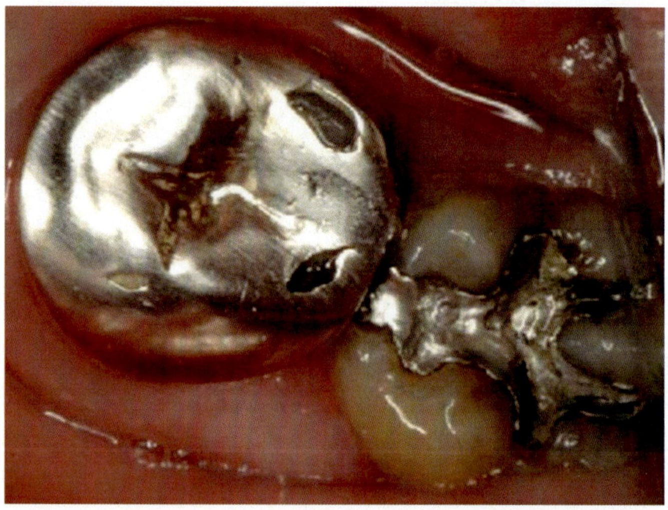

Fig. 3.88

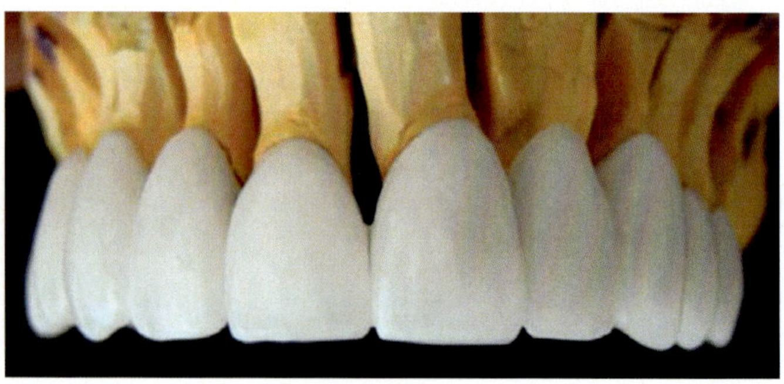

Fig. 3.89

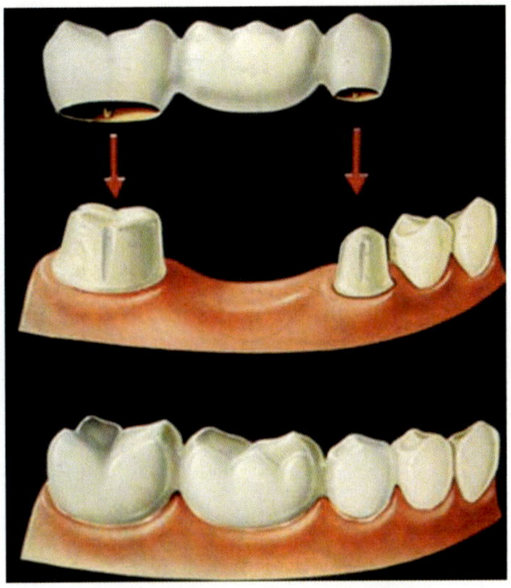

Fig. 3.90

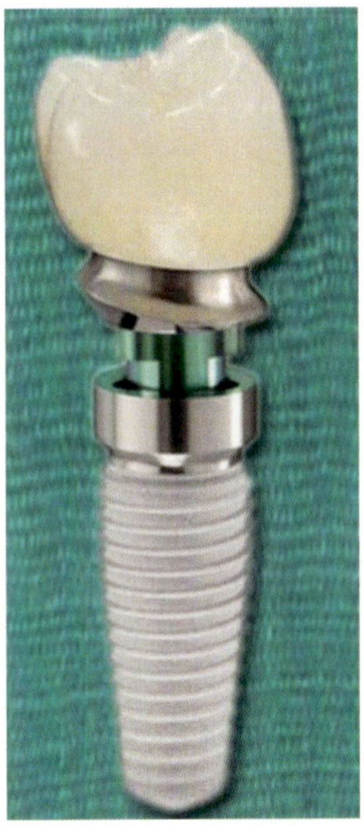

Fig. 3.91

- *Nonmetallic restorations:* Acrylics, silicates, composites, porcelain, partial and full removal prostheses.

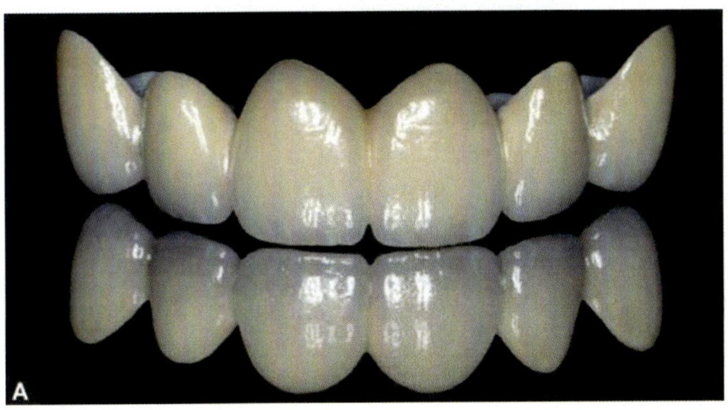

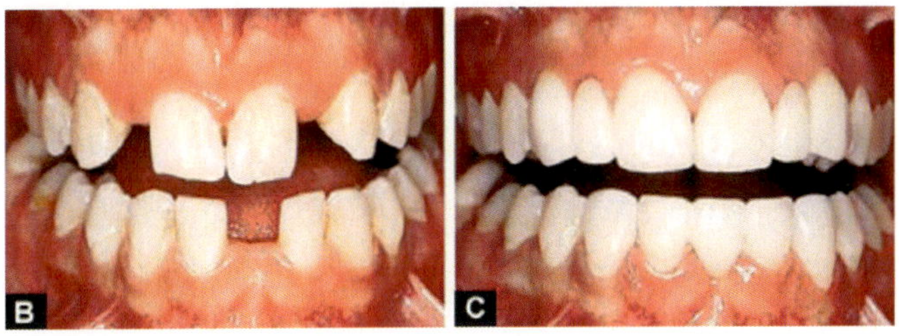

Figs 3.92A to C

Periodontium

Gingiva

Morphology/Pathology

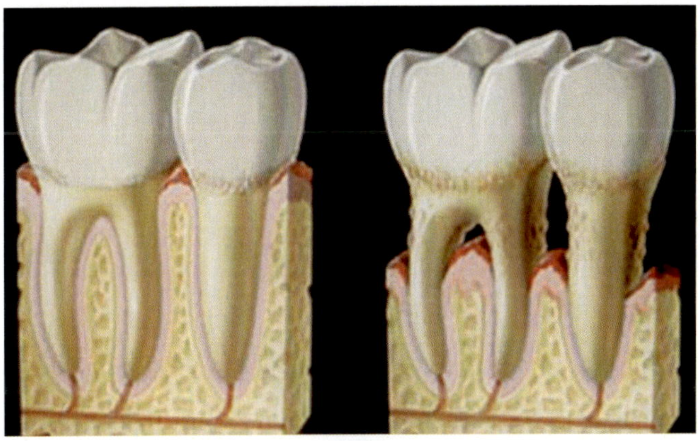

Fig. 3.93

Contour

Gingival recession, focal/diffuse enlargements

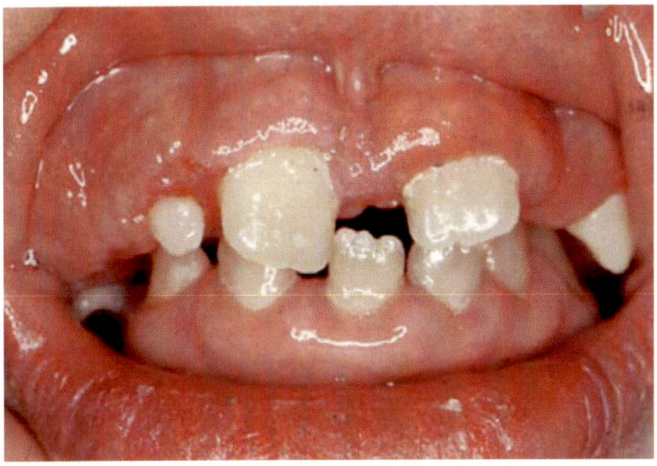

Fig. 3.94

Color

Inflammatory changes, physiologic or pathologic pigmentations, plaque oral hygiene status, stains, calculus.

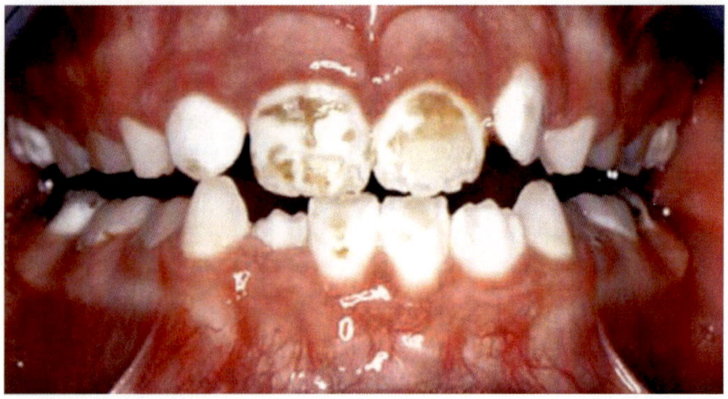

Fig. 3.95

Periodontal Ligament

Morphology/pathology, thickness, widening, lateral periodontal cyst. Alveolar process and lamina dura, height/contour/density of crestal bone, thickness of inter-radicular alveolar bone, exostoses, tori, pattern of lamina dura (loss, increased density), periodontal bone loss, trabecular bone pattern osteoporosis, radio-densities, residual root fragments, metallic fragments.

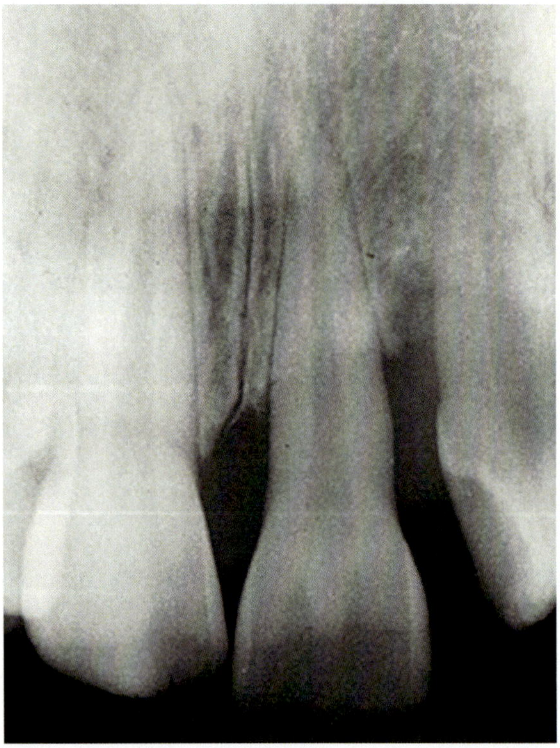

Fig. 3.96

MAXILLA AND MANDIBLE

Maxillary Sinuses

- Size, shape, retention cyst, antrolith, foreign bodies, oro antral fistula, relationship to adjacent teeth.

Anterior nasal spine, incisive canal, median palatal suture, incisive canal

Size, shape, cyst

Pterygoid Hamulus

Size, shape, fracture

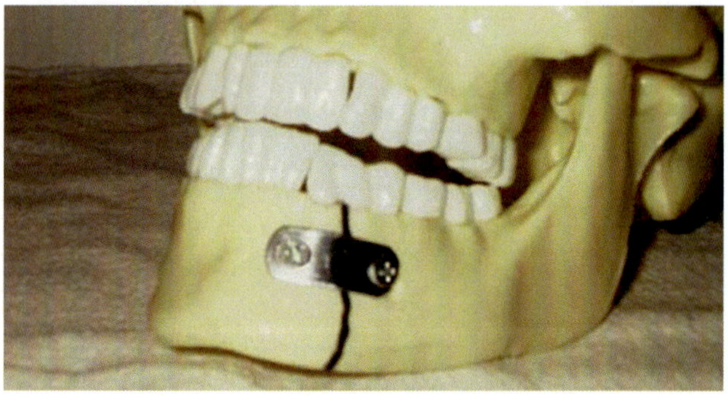

Fig. 3.97

Mandibular Canal/Mental Foramen

Diameter, anomalous (bifurcated), canal, relationship to adjacent teeth

Coronoid and Condylar Process

Size and shape

Temporomandibular Joint

Size, shape, hypertrophy/atrophy, ankylosis, fracture, arthritic changes

Other Pathologic Processes/Jaw Bones

Developmental/fissural cysts, hemorrhagic (traumatic) bone cyst, salivary gland depression, reactive neoplastic lesons, metabolic bone disease, other disorders inducing focal or diffuse radiolucencies or radiopacities, evidence of orthognathic surgery, or prior evidence of trauma (e.g. wire sutures, surgical pins, etc.)

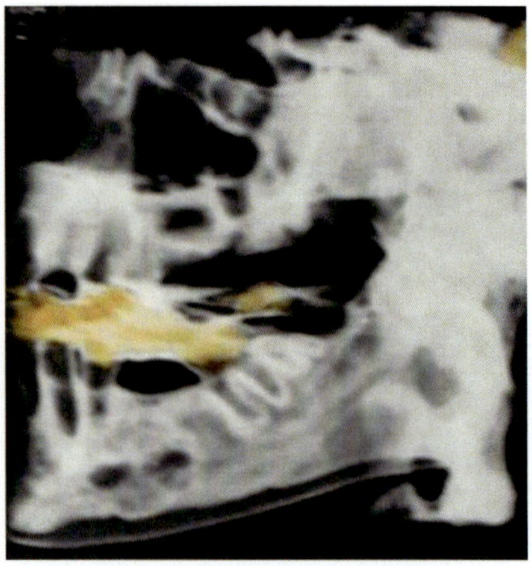

Fig. 3.98

CATEGORIES AND TERMINOLOGY FOR BODY IDENTIFICATION

Positive Identification

The antemortem and postmortem data match in sufficient detail to establish that they are from the same individual. In addition, there are no irreconcilable discrepancies.

Possible Identification

The antemortem and postmortem data have consistent features, but, due to the quality of either the postmortem remains or the antemortem evidence, it is not possible to positively establish dental identification.

Insufficient Evidence

The available information is insufficient to form the basis for a conclusion.

Exclusion

The antemortem and postmortem data are clearly inconsistent. However, it should be understood that identification by exclusion is a valid technique in certain circumstances.

Note: The forensic dentist is not ordinarily in a position to verify that the antemortem records are correct as to name, date, etc. ; therefore, the report should state that the conclusions are based on records which are purported to represent a particular individual.

Examination of the Case

- Examination of the victim is of utmost importance in forensic odontology. The evidences, which are the essential instruments for a forensic odontologist, should be collected and inspected with maximum care. Two forensic odontologists should examine, record and verify the findings to reduce misinterpretations. Examination of the victim or remains must be comprehensive incorporating all the available findings, however small it may be. It is carried out as in a living patient. A standard chart or odontogram is used to record the data. This will help to regularize the findings, especially where there are more than one victims. Comparisons can be done easily where they are needed, if all the data are recorded in a standard chart.
- Before making entry of examination findings information regarding the date and time of examination, name and designation of the person requesting for the examination, circumstances of the death, locus of the remains, names of the odontologists, names of the witnesses and gross physical description of the remains, etc., should be noted. All these are important from the view point of law.
- A systematic and comprehensive examination of teeth and soft tissues should be carried out. Although the same order as given, may not be followed, all these should be included.

Dentition

Complete charting of dentition using FDI system, or any other system followed, should be done. Whatever system is used, the findings should be understandable to others who are examining it. In the case of missing teeth, establishment of time of teeth loss is necessary. All characteristics like destruction by fire, presence of fillings, features of dentures, etc. should be noted down.

The characteristics of loss of teeth at various times are:

- *Postmortem loss:* In this case, the teeth were present at death but were lost subsequently. Postmortem teeth loss usually involved the single rooted teeth and the sockets of those teeth will have sharp margins without fractures.

Dentist	Last exam date
Address	Dentist contacted by Phone chart entered by Fax chart entered by
Surgery telephone Actual dental records	Chart checked against
Home telephone	Radiographs available?

- *Perimortem loss:* Those teeth that were lost at or very near the time of death are included under this type.
- *Premortem loss:* Teeth that may have been lost several hours or days prior to death constitute this group.
- A diagnosis of prior premortem loss may be confirmed by histologic examination of the soft tissues to confirm the presence of vital reaction to injury or the initiation of healing response. Abnormalities in shape, size, color, fractures and regreesive changes in the teeth are noted.

Effect of Fire on Tooth

In a fire, the gas in the intestines, stomach and lungs may cause the tongue to protrude and swell which usually protects the teeth from damage. If heat is applied slowly, the teeth are remarkably resistant to it. When heated severely and suddenly they may disintegrate immediately.

When heat is applied on bone, the crystals of bone will fuse resulting in shrinkage. Amalgam fillings may remain intact till 915°C, gold alloys melt above 915°C and procelain may survive till 1090°C. (Temperature changes on teeth)

Temp (°C)	*Effect on tooth*
100	– Mottled appearance of the crown and root appears light yellow.
200	– Crown and root appears orange color.
215	– Carbonization of pulp.
250	– Globular destruction of enamel.
300	– Yellowish-brown color crown, cracks appear in enamel, roots are destroyed and appear dark brown.
400	– Black-brown coloured crown with multiple cracks, crowns split.
500	– Enamel separates from the crown.
800	– Reduction in the volume of tooth and carbonization of the dentine.

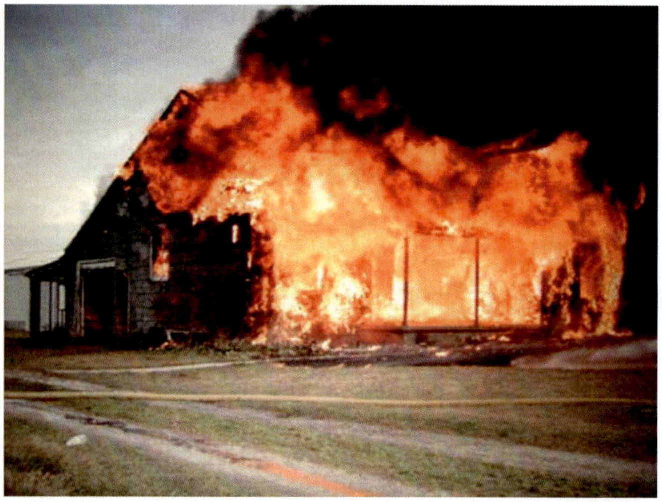

Fig. 3.99

Restorations and Prosthesis

- Restored teeth with the type of material used, surfaces involved by the restoration along with drawing of pattern of restoration should be noted. With the advent of tooth colored composite restorations it has become difficult to identify the restorations. Radiographs, ultraviolet light, infrared light and dyes are used for this purpose. An alternative light source such as polilight may be utilized for detecting composite and glass ionomer fillings. Burning destroys optical properties of glass ionomer, so it will be easy to identify a glass ionomer restoration.
- In a case of murder, porcelain fragment at the site of murder and porcelain fragment from the suspect were examined using scanning electron microscopy which demonstrated similarity in structure and air bubbles produced during baking process in both the samples, leading to identification. This incident demonstrates the importance of careful examination of the victim and the surroundings, in forensic odontology, for identifying the victim and, as in this case, culprit. Complete dentures, partial dentures, crown and bridges should be looked for type of materials used and the identification marks. The following methods can be used to place identification marks in dental prostheses.

Cast Gold Crowns and Metal Partial Dentures

- Under surface can be engraved with a bur or writing instrument with carbide tip.
  Acrylic dentures: Type the identification mark on paper or nylon or linen and insert it in the denture base before final closure.
  Injection-molded dentures: After processing the denture, place the identification mark typed on paper and cover it with self cure acrylic. If the patient objects to the above procedures a ballpoint pen with fluorescent ink can be used on pink tissue paper and included into the acrylic denture. This will show-up under ultraviolet light. The identification marks can be either the particulars of the patient or of the dentist or it can even be the singature of the laboratory where it has been made. For easy identification, any of the above type of markings has to be made on the dental appliances while fabricating it. Markings made on an appliance has to be standardized.
- It is not difficult to establish the identity between a partial denture and the jaw by comparing the number of missing teeth and the fit of the retainer to the abutment teeth. In the case of complete dentures found near skelatonized body it is difficult to establish the identity. Demonstration of the identity between the morphologic character of the denture base and the surface of the jaw bones may help to establish the identity. Minaguchi et al have described a superimposition method by taking a photograph of plaster model of the jaw with denture and placing a transparent photograph of plaster model to compare the arrangement of artificial teeth to the crest of the alveolar ridge.
- Periodontal status, signs of soft tissue and bony pathology, Angle's classification of occlusion alongwith overjet and overbite must be recorded in the odontogram. At this point extraoral, intraoral photographs, radiographs and impressions of dental arches should be made. Details about photographs, radiographs, etc. will be dealt with later in the book.

Collection of Antemortem Records

Successful identification depends on the existence of complete antemortem records so that comparison with postmortem data is possible. It is the duty of forensic dentist to collect all available records regarding the patients which includes dental charts, radiographs, photographs and models. Whenever, possible he should examine the original records and films because there is always loss of detail and resolution in the duplicates. Several antemortem records of the same person may be submitted from different dental practices for comparison. So all the details should be recharted and labeled as the "antemortem record".

Procedure of Identification

- Once the completed ante and postmortem records are available, the comparison analysis can begin. To establish identity, features present in the mouth must match that of antemortem records without inexplicable discrepancies.
- Apart from dental restorations, missing teeth, morphologic characters of teeth, racial characteristics of teeth, periodontal condition, oral habits, occupational marks, configuration of frontal sinuses, mastoid air spaces, sutural patterns, sella turcica, previous fractures, tori may also help in identification. Special methods such as chieloscopy, rugoscopy may also help.
- An inexplicable or irreconcilable discrepancy would exclude the identity. For example, if the antemortem record shows missing tooth which is present in the postmortem record. But the reverse may not exclude identification because the patient could have had a tooth extracted and records were not obtained.

Requirements for Positive Dental Identification

The quantity or quality of information necessary for determining positive dental identification has not been established. Keiser-Nielsen has suggested atleast twelve concordant dental features must be observed before an identification can be made. A lesser number may be needed if there are "extraordinary" concordant features. Example of this may include supernumerary or impacted tooth or an dental implant with identification mark.

Result of Identification Analysis

Result after comparison of records may be one of the following:

Positive Identification

Positive identification may be made on the existing evidence or by comparing ante and postmortem records. Finger prints and dental state provide most reliable points of identification than identification of personal belongings.

Presumptive (Possible) Identification

There are commonalities among comparable items in the antemortem and postmortem data; however, enough information may be missing from either source to prevent the establishment of a positive identification.

Insufficient Identification

There is insufficient supportive evidence available to compare and arrive at a conclusion based on scientific principles.

Exclusion of Identification

There are either explainable or unexplainable discrepancies among comparable items in the antemortem and postmortem databases resulting in inconsistencies that prevent the establishment of any identification.

Problems Associated with Dental Identification

- Identification of children is difficult because there may be scant or non-existent antemortem dental records. To overcome this special attention has to be paid regarding restorations, pit and fissure sealants, enamel hypoplasia, dental caries and abnormal sizes, shape or number of teeth, e.g. peg lateral, mesio dens, etc.
- If radiographs are not available, photographs of the child may aid to identify prominent features in the anterior teeth, e.g. spacing between teeth and rotated tooth, etc.
- Some of the other problems that may be seen when dental evidence is used for identification are listed below:
  - Lack of antemortem data
  - Insufficient information in the record
  - Errors in the ante or postmortem records
  - Inconsistencies between ante and postmortem datas
  - Poor condition of recovered remains
  - Use of abbreviations for recording dental treatment notes.

REPORT OF FORENSIC FINDINGS

When the comparison of antemortem and postmortem records is completed, a complete, understandable report is prepared. This report should include the following information.

- Medical examiner or coroner number
- Place of examination and comparison
- Date of examination and comparison
- Name, address, phone numbers of the forensic dentist.
- Tentative name of the victim (if known)
- Antemortem and postmortem charting
- Text report covering all of the points that matched if a positive identification is made or the inconsistencies and impossibilities if there is no match
- Name, address, phone numbers of the dentist who has provided the antemortem records
- The dentist needs to consider the necessary equipment for a complete postmortem examination. The following list includes some equipment that is supplied by the dentist and some that usually is available in the mortuary:
  - Examination gloves
  - Disposable mask
  - Eye protection/magnification loupes
  - Dental mirror
  - Dental explorers
  - Forceps, curved and straight

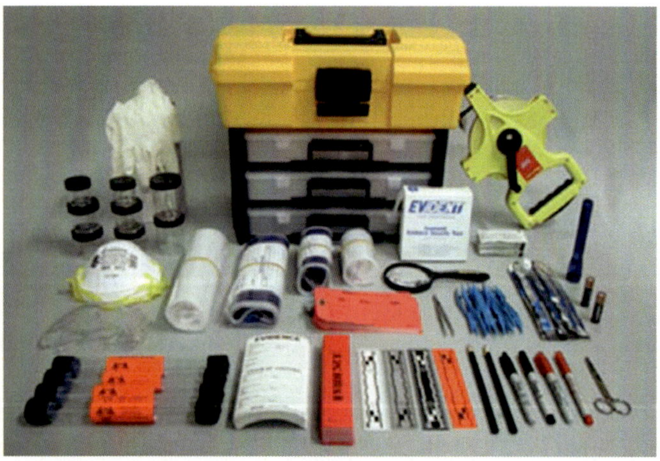

Fig. 3.100

- Other dental hand instruments
- Minnesota retractor
- Tooth brushes
- Denture brush
- Radiograph holders
- View box
- Camera, lenses, flash
- Photomirrors
- Plastic lip retractors
- Molt mouth prop

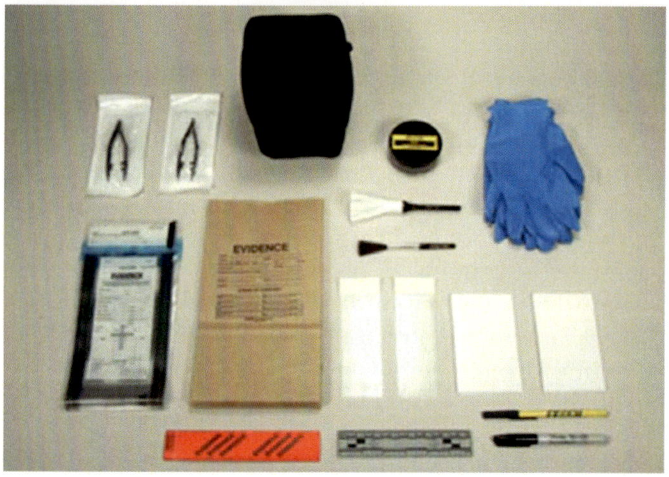

Fig. 3.101

- Mouth props (rubber)
- Pens, pencils, notepaper
- Examination forms
- Dental radiographic film

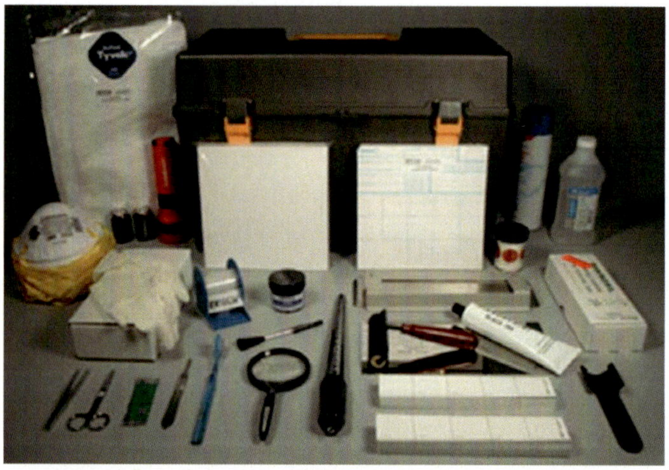

Fig. 3.102

- Transillumination light
- Head lamp

Although the forensic odontologist is responsible for the oral and dental examination of the deceased, the parameters of such an examination should be established with the Medical Examiner. In some cases. it is necessary to excise facial tissues or to remove the maxilla, mandible, or both to gain access to the dentition. Such dissections never should take place without the expressed concurrence of the pathologist. To ensure that there are no misunderstandings about the type of examination or comparison requested, it may be helpful to use a written consultation request form similar to that used in hospitals for soliciting consultation from other specialists to aid in a patient's care.

Positive Identification

There is a sufficient match between antemortem and postmortem data to establish that they are from the same individual. There are no unexplained discrepancies.

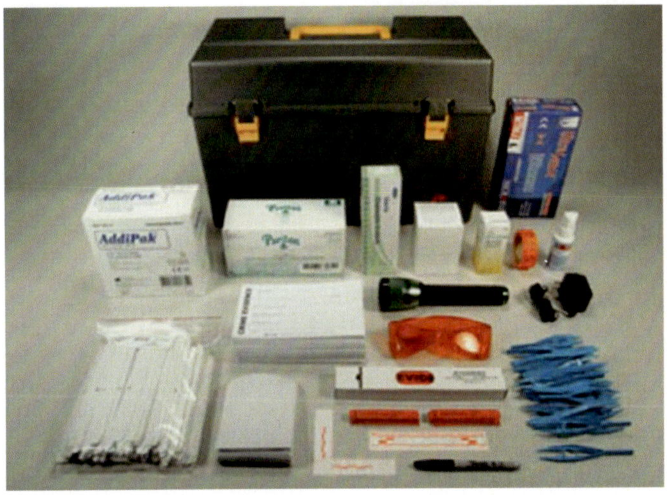

Fig. 3.103

Possible Identification

There are consistent features between antemortem and postmortem data, but because of poor-quality records antemortem and postmortem data, missing postmortem information, a positive identification cannot be established.

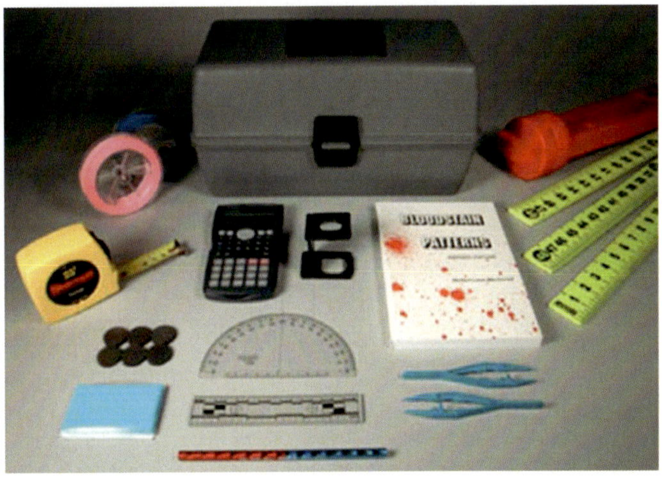

Fig. 3.104

Insufficient Evidence

The information available is not adequate to make a reasonable conclusion.

Exclusion

There are clear (unexplainable) inconsistencies between the antemortem and postmortem data.

CHAPTER 4

Dental Team

INTRODUCTION

- Dental teams have been a major part in disaster mass fatality response for many years and continue to be an essential part of responses to more recent incidents.
- A disaster is a sudden occurrence that exceeds the resources available in a community to deal with it. A mass fatality incident is an occurrence that causes loss of life that exceeds death investigation resources in a community. As part of response, added resources are offered by agencies outside the normal community response agencies. A disaster contingency plan identifies and develops plans to use such resources should the need arise. The dental team is a good example of such a resource because the team can be developed and trained as a unit to be ready if needed.

INCIDENT COMMAND

PIO	Safety Officer		
Liaison Officer	Legal Officer		
Operations	Planing	Logistics	Finance

- Site Operations Branch—security, search and recovery, investigative, decontamination
- Mortuary Services Branch—morgue operations, identification, disposition
- Family Assistance Branch—facility unit, family support, interview

INCIDENT COMMAND SYSTEM (ICS)

- There are two types of dental identification teams—the traditional locally based teams and the newer dental teams integrated into the disaster mortuary operational response team (DMORT) system.
  - The traditional dental team for response to a mass fatality incident has been the community-based or state-based dental identification team, many of which are sponsored by state dental associations. The teams often are led by the chief forensic dentist, who works with the local medical examiner or coroner. Team members include dentists, hygienists, and dental assistants.
  - A second type of team emerging and being used increasingly is the DMORT. The DMORT is a part of the National Disaster Medical System under the US Department of Public Health. A DMORT team consists of a dental team, forensic pathology team, anthropology and laboratory support, photographic and communication support, logistics team, and mortuary science team. The federal government funds the DMORT, and team members are selected for their expertise to become temporary federal emergency employees.

GUIDELINES FOR THE DEVELOPMENT OF A DISASTER DENTAL IDENTIFICATION TEAM

History

- Natural or man made catastrophes often result in multiple casualties under circumstances that make their identification difficult. It has long been recognized that under these circumstances, the use of dental records and X-rays by a team of trained forensic odontologists can greatly assist in the expeditious identification of the casualties. This facilitation of the identification and release of the victims to their families, not only provides a humanitarian service relieving the feelings suffering and helplessness, but also satisfies several medicolegal requiremetns. It is only a matter of time, when and where a mass disaster will occur.
- Based upon the significant role that forensic odontology has played in recent disaster response, it is the goal of the American Board of Forensic Odontology. Inc. to make available, to all who may have need, a simple but complete set of guidelines for the development of a dental identification team. Formal documentation of death demands positive identification. The degree of success in any disaster investigation is directly porportional to the degree of preparation.

Purpose

These guidelines are designed as a resource for those agencies or jurisdictions who wish to develop an identification team either as a free standing unit or as a section of an overall disaster preparedness plan for a specific region. Realizing no two disasters are identical, nor that the needs of all jurisdictions are the same, modification of any plan may be necessary. Based upon the combined experience of many Diplomates with first hand experience in the identification of multiple casualties, these guidelines are flexible. They provide a complete, but simple outline around which an organization can develop and identification team to suit its purposes.

Team Development

- Basic to any disaster identification team plan is the development of a concept of operation. How will your team function? Many states have organized dental identification teams, some under the auspieces of their state dental societies. The Council on Dental Practice of the American Dental Association has taken on the task of assisting and coordinating the activity. Will your team be integrated into an overall Emergency Government Plan for an entire state, or will it serve a country or region? Will your team be a part of a Disaster Mortuary Team (DMORT), under the National Disaster Medical Service?
- If trained odontologists are not available to form the core of the team, how will the training be accomplished? Will the team be dependent upon assistant from odontologists from other areas, or will it be free standing with capability of handling all of it's own functions? Once some of these questions are answered, those who are organizing the team can begin to consider the development of a plan, based upon four general areas:
  - Team personnel
  - Team organization
  - Equipment and supplies
  - Safety and health considerations.

Facilities

- There is overlap between the odontologists, pathologists and funeral directors in the need for some of the equipment and supplies. Some of the equipment may be available from these sources and used jointly.
- Outline of a team organization
- Initial organizational planning
- Evaluate your need for a dental identification team
- Responsibility to the public
- Probability of an incident
- Prior existence of area or state teams
- Evaluate resources
- Trained dental personnel
- Equipment and supplies
- Financial assistance
- State and local dental societies
- State and local emergency management agencies
- Organizational implementation
- Team leadership
- Written organizational plan
- Written participation agreement
- Written protocol with job descriptions
- Flow chart for division of duties
- Written record of participation and training
- Sponsorship
- State Dental Association
- State Emergency Government Administration
- State or local Medical Examiner/Coroner
- Team personnel
- Source
- Diplomates of the American Board of Forensic Odontology
- Qualified odontologists
- A nucleus of highly trained odontologist's are necessary to serve in a supervisory and instructional capacity
- The remainder of the team may be composed of dental personnel with skills in dentistry and limited training in forensic dentistry
- Number of Personnel
- Consider your potential for a disaster and its size
- Major metropolitan area vs small city or rural area
- International Jetport vs local airport
- Presence of a geologic fault, volcano
- Reality of floods, hurricanes, or tornadoes
- Hazardous and explosive chemical industry
- Sources for personnel recruitment
- Forensic organizations
- Dental Societies
- Dental Schools
- Additional resources
- Armed Forces Institute of Pathology, Department of Oral Pathology
- National Disaster Medical Service, Disaster Mortuary Teams
- Odonotologists in Armed Forces Reserve Units.
- Training
- Initial training

- Courses are Offered by
  - Armed Forces Institute of Pathology
  - University Dental Schools, Continuing Education Courses
  - National and state dental society meetings

OTHER RESOURCES

- Fire and rescue services training locally
- Hazardous Materials Teams (HAZAT) training courses
- Cost of training
- Individual's responsibility
- Sponsoring organization's responsibility
- Emergency Government Funds
- Scheduling of periodic continuing education drills
- Quarterly would be very difficult
- Semiannually is possible
- Yearly is probably the most realistic
- Cross training of section members is highly desirable
- Objectives of training
- Familiarity with subject
- Understanding dental identification
- Antemortem problems and procedures
- Acquiring flight manifests and names
- Locating and securing dental records
- Problems with poor quality records
- Postmortem problems and procedures
- Gaining access to dental structures
- Obtaining postmortem radiographs
- Fragmentation and commingling
- Comparison section problems
- Coping with large numbers of records
- Computer vs manual searches
- Identification of fragmented and commingled remains
- Determination of the number of the team members required
- Based upon magnitude of disaster
- The condition of the human remains
- Based upon the estimated time required
- Special skills required
- Dentists with forensic training, oral surgeons, oral pathologists
- Auxiliary personnel, hygienists, assistants for records compilation
- Computer-assisted identification program specialists
- Psychologists trained in critical incident stress disorder (CISD)
- An experienced member to serve as a liaison with other sections of the investigative team
- Amateur radioservice operators for emergency communications
- Clergy
- Staging area
- Location
- Transportation of team personnel to the morgue site
- Private vehicles
- Buses, vans or four-wheel drive vehicle
- Access to the disaster area by dental personnel for the recovery of fragmentary dental evidence
- Legal considerations
- Status of the team members as volunteers or employees
- Responsibility for their health and safety
- Worker's compensation or liability insurance to cover any injury or exposure
- Compensation of the team members
- Rate
- Establishment of the rate according to experience, training and skill
- Responsibility for the time and record keeping
- Agency or underwriter responsible for payment
- Team members should be informed of their probable compensation prior to participation
- Consider a written agreement for team members
- Rules and regulations for participation
- Authorized photography
- Authorized press interviews only by official spokesperson
- Procedure for activation and participation
- Responsibilities.
- Participation in continuing education
- Obligation to report changes in telephone number or address
- Code of ethics
- Nondisclosure of privileged information
- Report to staging area only when activated
- No unauthorized contact with the media
- Written authorization from Coroner or Medical Examiner to conduct a limited autopsy
- Methods to gain access to the teeth
- Viewable vs nonviewable cases
- Specific authorization on removal of jaws
- Written authorization for the retention of any tissue
- Jurisdictional consideration
- Conflict of any of the identification team guidelines with an existing emergency government disaster plan
- Limitation of the team's area of operation
- State or governmental licensure considerations applicable
- Mutual aid agreements already in effect for other dental identification teams
- Mobilization procedure (activation)
- Method for both drills and actual notification
- Phone
- FAX

- One individual solely responsible for placing all calls for activation is recommended
- Ability to confirm the team member's availability
- Ascertain the duration of assignment the team member can accept
- Assign a specific time to report or duty to be performed
- Periodic update of telephone contact numbers and phone drill
- Annually should be the minimum to keep records current
- More frequently is desirable
- Determination of which team members are to be activated
- Decided by the team leader, or designee, in consultation with the Medical Examinar.

Examiner/Coroner and Based Upon

- Number of fatalities
- Skills required
- Security/Identification of Authorized Team Personnel
- Photoidentification cards are most fool proof
- Distinctive color baseball caps with logo identify from a distance
- Distinctive colored protective equipment, e.g. vests are especially valuable at the disaster site
- Team organization/structure
- Can be divided into sections for specific training and duties
- Antemortem records section
- Postmortem, photography and X-ray section
- Comparison section
- Size of sections determined by magnitude of catastrophe
- Team leader, alternate team leader and section supervisors should be on call 24 hours at a time to effectively be able to activate the team
- Units of the team can be organized regionally
- Equipment and supplies
- Basic equipment
- Dental X-ray machine(s)
- Auto film processor(s) with daylight loader
- Autopsy equipment (much may be available from Medical Examiner or Coroner office)
- Bard parker handles and blades
- Rib cutters
- Long handle pruning shears
- Gurneys and tables
- Lighting (may be available from emergency government)
- Photographic equipment
- Computer hardware/software — (useful for large numbers of fatalities)
- Copy machine(s) and paper
- Consider having a backup available for all equipment
- Immediate availability of supplies and equipment
- Prior arrangements in place with potential suppliers are essential.
- Evening, weekend and holiday contact numbers are a necessity. Disaster can strike anytime
- Consider an alternate source just in case
- Advance financial arrangements eliminate the need for cash at the time of procurement
- Annual review of equipment needs and contact numbers of personnel authorized to provide emergency use of the equipment to provide the supplies must be accomplished
- Supplies (Exact items required and quantity will be determined by the individual team resources and needs. Remember some supplies have a limited shelf life and mut be replaced periodically.
- Dental X-ray film and mounts/photographic film
- Dental charts (standardized format), manila envelopes, magic markers and colored pencils
- Rubber gloves (heavy duty), rubber aprons and face masks and shields or eye protection
- Protective footwear (rubber boots)
- Banker boxes for files
- The quantity of supplies is driven by the number of casualties
- Foot locker or storage boxes for small equipment
- Responsibility for cleaning and sterilizing instruments and returning instruments and equipment.
- Responsibility for restocking supplies used
- Consider the other agencies involved in the disaster response as a resource for coordination of the procurement of equipment and supplies.
- Medical Examiner or Coroner offices
- National Funeral Directors Association Mobile Disaster Mortuary
- Fire and Rescue Services
- Emergency Government Coordinators
- Clean-up, storage and restocking of equipment and supplies
- Cleaning and sterilization of equipment can be accomplished by local hospitals as a public service or Medical Examiner facilities.
- Storage location between disaster response (must be accessible at all times)
- Airport warehouse facility
- Emergency Government facility
- Medical Examiner Office
- Responsibility for restocking supplies
- Coroner/Medical Examiner
- Emergency Government Office-Country, State, National-Federal Emergency Management Agency.
- The identification team

- Safety and Health of Team Members must be considered.
- Team leaders must be aware of their responsibilities
- Team teaders and teampersonnel must be properly trained and aware of
  - Radiologic hazards
  - Bloodborne pathogens
  - Toxic chemicals
  - Hazardous sharp debris
  - Team member must receive biologic hazard and blood borne pathogens training annually and be documented.
  - A written plan and record of periodic training must be maintained
  - Avoid long hours or shifts
  - Increase in critical incident stress
  - Increase in mistakes and accidents
  - Doesn't allow for adequate cleaning of the morgue site

IMMUNIZATION

- Tetanus
- Hepatitis B
- Special situation immunizations for foreign locations
- Cost borne by the sponsoring organization
- Records should be kept and updated per OSHA regulations
- A custodian of these records must be designated
- Protective gear for personnel is a necessity
- Team members must be trained in the use of this equipment
- Protective equipment must be immediately available
- Agency responsible for providing the protective equipment

STORAGE LOCATION

- Responsibility for disbursing/maintaining it
- Psychological debriefing and counseling should be available. Since this is a situation common to all disaster workers, it ordinarily is not the responsibility of the dental identification team to arrange for this service. However, dental team members should be aware that their work can be psychologically taxing.
- Access to experts in post-traumatic stress counseling
- Access to clergy
- Facilities
- Although this is responsibility of the Coroner or Medical Examiner, many smaller jurisdictions have never experienced a catastrophe involving mass fatalities. It should, therefore, be considered by the experienced dental identification team, since they may provide valuable advice
- Adequate temporary morgue sites must be selected in advance
- All Coroner/Medical Examiner offices do not have a written disaster plan in place, so potential sites may not be in place
- Experienced odontologists may be able to assist them in developing this plan, because of their prior experience.
- In general, it is advantageous to plan for the use of existing facilities to their maximum before setting-up a temporary morgue.
- Alternate sites also should be considered as a back-up
- Sanitation facilities must be available at all of the potential sites
- Hot running water and soap, toilets and toilet paper
- Arrangements for food and a rest area for team members
- Sources for food and drink
- Salvation Army Canteen
- Red cross volunteers
- Volunteers
- Service clubs
- Church groups
- Consider the maximum length of time a team member should work
- This work is stressful
- Be aware of post traumatic stress disorder
- Provide for mandatory periodic breaks and rotate duties
- Rest in an area removed from the morgue is essential
- Consider rotating team members between sections frequently
- Provide chairs or stools for use of team members while working
- Standard working hours are the least stressful.
- Immediate reservation of blocks of hotel or motel rooms by the office of emergency government, or other authorized agency, for the use of disaster personnel is necessary to prevent the media from typing up all of the rooms available for miles around.
- Area perimeter security is the responsibility of the ranking law enforcement official present. However, the dental team must be aware of the necessity for perimeter security and be readily identified.
- Protection of personal effects of victims
- Excluding the curious and unauthorized
- Prevention of unauthorized photography by the media
- Can be provided by governmental or private agencies.
- Working in shifts, around the clock, is to be avoided, unless absolutely necessary. The use of adequately cross-trained supervisory personnel is mandatory.

CHAPTER 5

Examination Methods

INTRODUCTION

Radiographs being nondestructive method play a vital role in forensive dentistry to uncover the hidden facts which can't be seen by means of physical examination. They have helped to solve difficult cases in the forensic science.

USES

Identification of Victims

- Radiographs are helpful to determine age of an individual by assessing the stage of eruption of teeth.
- Skull radiographs can be used in identification by superimposing an antemortem radiographs or photographs. Since frontal sinuses are known for greatest normal variations among individuals they are used for this purpose. Racial variations among individuals are used for this purpose. Racial variations in the configuration of frontal sinuses are also seen. Yoshino et al have classified frontal sinuses based on size, bilateral asymmetry, superiority of side, outline of upper borders, presence of partial septa and supra orbital cells and reported a criminal case in which frontal sinus was used to identify a person.
- Sassouni has suggested use of measurements in posteroanterior and lateral radiographs of the skull to match the ante and postmortem radiographs, which includes
  - Bigonial width
  - Cranial height (from mastoid to vertex)
  - Bimaxillary breadth
  - Height from bigonial width to temporal crest
  - Maximum cranial breadth
  - Frontal sinus breadth
  - Incisor height
  - Facial height.

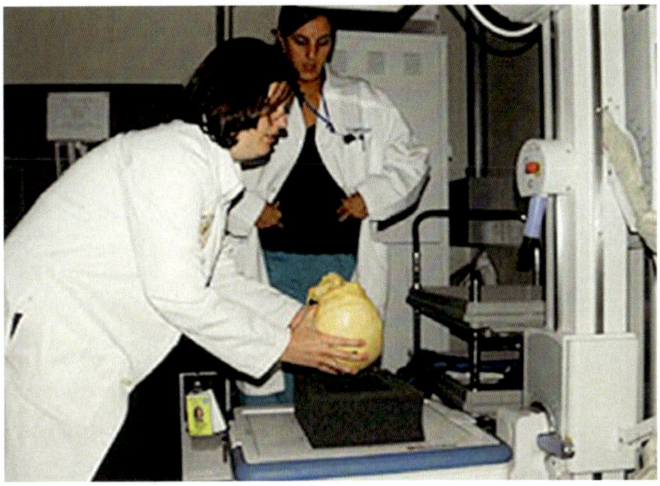

Fig. 5.1

Uses of Dental Radiographs in Identification

- Dental radiographs may be compared from ante and postmortem records for congenital and acquired abnormalities such as malformed tooth, caries, restorations, root canal fillings, etc. Law et al have injected radiopaque substances into the sockets of skeletonized remains to reconstruct the root canal morphology to compare with antemortem radiographs.
- A new method using digital subtraction image analysis of bitewing radiographs provided reliable registration for positive identity when certain criteria were used.
- Age of the extraction socket can be determined from the appearance of the socket in the radiograph.

First evidence of healing	→	Fuzziness of lamina dura due to resorption
Early stages after extraction	→	Granular appearance of the socket due to new bone formation
Late stages	→	Normal trabecular bone pattern.

Evidence in the Identification of Suspect

- Cases have been reported where suspects were identified because of fractured tooth parts of victims in the body of the suspects or fractured tooth of suspect in the victim as in the bite mark cases.
- Deliberate alterations in the shape of the teeth in suspects can be identified with radiographs in bite mark cases.

Determine the Cause of Death

Radiographs may provide evidence of bullets or foreign bodies in the soft tissues following fire arm incidents and explosions. After air crash accidents the cause of crash may be elucidated by the presence of radiopaque objects in the soft tissues. This is due to contamination with molten aircraft metal producing irregular shaped radiopacity.

Find Faulty Charting of Teeth

Sometimes while charting postmortem data teeth may be wrongly numbered especially in cases where adjacent tooth migrate into the extraction space. This can be corrected using radiographs.

Basic Principle Used for Postmortem Radiograph

When a radiograph of postmortem remains is performed to compare with antemortem radiograph "identical projection" must be achieved with similar magnification, exposure factors and angulation so as to reproduce the antemortem radiograph like image. This job is carried out by using various angles of projection and by varying technical factors.

General Considerations

Radiographs should be taken before and after head and neck autopsy. Whenever possible, radiographs should be made at the scene of accident or crime. They should be properly labeled with identification number, site and date of examination for future reference. All intra and exraoral projections including panoramic radiographs have to be taken as and when it is needed depending on the case and type of remains.

Intraoral Radiographs

- Intraoral radiographs are difficult to perform particularly when there is restricted mouth opening. It may be necessary to remove soft tissues from the floor of the mouth or cheeks to insert the film. A miniature intraoral X-ray source may be used.
- Resected maxilla may be split through the midpalatal suture. The posterior mandible and maxilla are placed on occlusal film to produce an "enlarged bite-wing film".
- Whenever fragmented remains consisting of teeth, restorations, bone pieces, appliances are recovered, they have to be separated by the method proposed by Johanson.

Johanson's Method

- Place the debris on a plastic grid.
- Place the film on a wire grid identical to the plastic grid.
- From the resultant radiograph type of remain can be identified.

TECHNICAL FACTORS

Sources of X-ray

Intraoral source: Radioactive Iodine 125 can be used to expose the radiograph. It emits 27.4 keV X-rays. It is expensive and has a short half life of 60 days. Advantage of this source is that it eliminates the need for jaw resection for the purpose of taking radiographs as it can be introduced into the oral cavity with trocar and cannula.

Extraoral source: Extraoral source of X-rays are provided from dental or medical X-ray machines.

Film Holder

Films are held in position with hemostats, tapes or gauze stuffed in the mouth or using modeling clay.

EXPOSURE FACTORS

- Exposure time depends on the density of the object. Density increases with soft tissues and skull recovered from the water, but decreases due to fire. Usually exposure time should be reduced to one half to two thirds of normal exposure for remains with soft tissue. Skeletonized remains need only one half of the normal exposure.
- To differentiate tooth and filling MA should be reduced with increased exposure time. Generally, films should be repeated with varying KVP, mA and exposure time.

Films

Slower films are used in forensic cases to enhance the details. Double film pockets eliminate the need for duplication. For extraoral radiographs slow films and intensifying screens should be used.

Processing

- Best results can be obtained with manual processing using "visual method" to adjust and reproduce films resembling antemortem films.
- All the radiographs should be duplicated and filed for future reference.

Improving the Bad Quality Radiographs

There are few methods which can be utilized to improve too dark or too light radiographs.

Chemical Method

Dark radiographs may be lightened by chemically removing some of the silver that forms the image and light films may be intensified by binding another visible substance to the silver.

Duplication Method

While duplicating a film by increasing or decreasing light exposure, radiographs can be made light or dark as required.

Photographic Method

Changing transmitted light intensity from a view box, altering exposure time or lens opening or using different speed photographic films radiographs can be photographed to overcome poor quality.

Electronic Imaging Techniques

- Computerized digital image processing and manipulation can enhance observer's ability to detect from defective radiographs.
- Andersen L, Wenzel A. Individual identification by means of conventional bite wing film and subtraction radiography. *Foren Sci Int* 1995;72:55-64.
- **Photographs** are important adjunct to the written records. If properly taken they are one of the most reliable and useful tools. Accuracy and reproducibility are of greatest important for use in forensic science.

Advantages

- Its clarity and comprehensibility helps to overcome language barriers. Relationships of size and shape can be depicted.
- Details can be recorded and studied later.
- Provides graphic evidence, which is often easy to understand than a detailed verbal description.
- Aids in the presentation of case in the court of law.

Uses in Forensic Dentistry

Photographs can be taken to record details of models, prosthesis, remains or resected jaws. It is extensively used in the bite mark analysis. Special photographic superimposition techniques aid in identification of unknown remains.

Photographic Superimposition Technique

- When the victims of decomposed skeletonized body have to be identified one of the method uses superimposition of the facial photograph or photograph of dentition of the victim over the skull. Most often this technique is not considered as reliable one because some adjustments are needed to bring antemortem photographs and postmortem photographs to the same size. But this method can be used along with other types of identification systems.
- First case to be identified using the photographic superimposition technique was in the year 1938 called as "Ruxton Case".
- If there are objects with known dimensions are present in the antemortem photographs (e.g.ornaments), it will be useful to enlarge the photograph of victims to true life size. If such articles are not seen then anatomical or anthropologic measurements of facial soft tissues can be used to obtain superimposition by best fit. McKenna et al have utilized measurements of visible portion of dentition to obtain true life size photograph of the object.

Photographic Superimposition of Teeth

- When a face is photographed teeth are often in focus. Thus the anterior teeth in the skull could provide a size determinant for the enlargement of the antemortem photograph. McKenna achieved hundred percent success in a blind trial by superimposition of photographs and plastic models of dentition of individuals.
- Facial aspect to teeth have a number of measurable features such as coronal angle, mesial and distal incisal angle, maximum width and height, etc. Contour profiles and special characters such as pitting, fractures and attrition may also aid in identification.
- Chandra H has discussed a case where the victim was identified by superimposing buccal occlusal line in the antemortem photograph and skull photograph.

Skull Superimposition Technique

Skull superimposition technique is done as described below:

Step 1: Skull should be photographed from the same orientation as that of the portraits selected for comparison. This can be achieved by using a skull holding device called "goniometer" which helps to record and reposition linear and angular measurements of the position of the camera relative to the skulls.

Step 2: By placing positive and negative skull photograph on transparent film a thin "line profile" is obtained.

Step 3: Using the identifiable land marks the line profile and antemortem photograph are superimposed. Look for the dimensions and matching between skull landmarks with land marks on the face (e.g. supraorbital ridge of the skull may be matched with eyebrow).

COMPUTERS

- The crash of the Arrow Air charter aircraft in Gander, Newfoundland on December 12, 1985, proved to be a landmark in the history of forensic odontology. Among other notable successes attained by the identification teams, the disaster successfully used a computerized identification system as part of the comparison process. This system, the **Computer Assisted Postmortem Identification System (CAPMI),** provided a simple user-friendly system with enough specificity to aid the dental identification team adequately. CAPMI grew to become the most widely used computer identification assistance program in the United States. Computers allow the storage of a large number of records, facilitate comparisons, and allow data to be shared easily between agencies.
- Descriptive information about teeth can be used to aid in the establishment of identification. Dental identifications rely on the comparison of dental charateristics. If data for dental information are limited to the restored surfaces, the placement of crowns, and the absence or presence of teeth, the resultant curve shows a bimodel distribution.
- The CAPMI system was developed by Lorton at the US Army Institute of Dental Research. Dental information had been shown to be vital to successful identification efforts in mass fatality situations. Dental information is useful because teeth resist trauma, and antemortem records exist for comparison. The goal of the program is to provide an effective matching program in terms of specificity, time and cost management.
- Principles used in the development of CAPMI are based on three areas of data management: Gathering the data, the comparison and selection process, and verification. Data gathering simplifies possible antemortem and postmortem data into similar usable forms.
- Teeth present numerous characteristics for comparison. CAPMI limits the primary characteristics to information on surfaces restored (MODEL or crown) and presence or absence of a tooth (V, X, U). This limiting of information eliminates subjectivity as much as possible.
- Computers have migrated from DOS-based operating systems to graphic user interfaces (GUIs) such as Windows. The Windows environment allows for greater ease of use, makes a wide array of device drivers available, and can display graphics readily.
- Win ID2 users can create new date collections called queries. Queries are formed using the data manipulation features of Microsoft Access. Queries are used to restrict data to records that fulfill certain criteria. An example of a query is a collection of all records of all African-American men from the antemortem table. A comparison could then be done to an unknown postmortem record. This feature is an excellent tool when using a large missing persons database. WinID was written to serve two purposes : (1) Missing person recovered body database formation and maintenance and (2) Mass disaster human identification. Both of these tasks are aided by WinID being able to sift through large amounts of data to generate a list of best matches. The best-match comparisons are generated from a key record compared with a target table or query.
- For the program to work, data must be processed and entered. A crucial task for the computer section of a dental identification team is to make the data collection and notation uniform among all involved.
- Postmortem data are developed from the recovered remains. The numbering of the remains conforms to the numbering system of overseeing agency, usually the Medical Examiner-Coroner. Using the composite postmortem charts, dental information is entered into the program. Guidelines cover whether or not material codes will be entered and how to manage sealants or dental anomalies. Guidelines cover how broken and fragmented teeth will be noted as well as how fragmented dental remains will be related to whole body recoveries. All entries should be verified.

- Antemortem record entry has several challenges. Records vary from complete to incomplete, and errors in charting are encountered. Interpretation of records and radiographs varies between examiners as to exactly which surfaces are restored. To conform to the ideal of placing all records into similar usable forms, the level of information must be the same. Guidelines for the antemortem record team are needed to standardize entries and to ensure an accurate database. Guidelines include such areas as third molar status, presence or absence of facial or lingual restorations, anomalies, notation of restorative materials, notation of sealants, and notation of caries. To simplify, it is recommended that only surfaces that can be verified be indicated to prevent mismatch.
- WinID uses tooth codes developed for CAPMI. The primary codes are basically surfaces restored and presence or absence of a tooth. They provide the basis for the comparison algorithm. Each tooth field must have at least one primary code. The secondary codes are modifiers, allowing entry of extra information for each tooth. The secondary codes are not used in the best-match comparison but can be used to limit a LOOK sort. The codes are listed in the accompanying box.

Table 5.1: WinID tooth codes

Primary codes	*Secondary codes*
U - Unerupted tooth	A - Abnormality
V - Virgin/unrestored tooth	B - Deciduous tooth
X - Missing/extracted tooth	E - Resin restorative
C - Crown	G - Gold restorative
J - Tooth fractured/ missing postmortem	H - Porcelain restorative
I - No information on status restorative	N - Nonprecious metal
M - Mesial	P - Pontic present
O - Occlusal	Q - Quarter crown
I - Incisal	R - Root canal filling
D - Distal	S - Amalgam restorative
F - Facial	T - Denture tooth present
L - Lingual restorative	Z - Caries or temporary

Table 5.2: Chart information form a dental record with written and graphic entries but no radiographs

Tooth #	*Antemortem record*	*Status*	*Code*
1	Marked as X on graphic chart	Missing or impacted	/
2	O am placed 92, F am placed 94, DOL am 95	MO-A, F-A, DOL-A	MODEL
3	RTC 95, PFM 96	PFM-CR, Endo	C-HR
4	Retained primary A, MO-composite 95	MO-CO, retained primary tooth	MO-BE (on tooth #4)
5	Unmarked on graphic chart	Unrestored	V
6	Chart notes impaction	Impacted	U
7	F-composite 94, L-alloy 94	F-CO, L-AM	FL-ES
8	ML composite 94, graphic chart shows MF	ML-CO or MF-CO	M-E

Tabel 5.3: Postmortem coding

Tooth #	*Postmortem status*	*Composite*	*Code*
26	Missing, socket present	PX (missing postmortem)	J
27	Crown fractured off, root present	Fractured	J
28	Crown prep evident, crown lost	Crown	C
29	Tooth missing, site healed	X, Pontic?	X
30	Crown prep, crown missing, endo and postcore present	CR, Endo, Post	C-R
31	MO amalgam, distal of tooth fixed with DO prep evident	MO-A, DO-?	MOD
32	Impacted with cyst	IMP	U-A

Comparisons are most often the comparison of dental remains received to the antemortem record database. This comparison process is done for each of the 32 tooth fields on the key record to each of the 32 tooth fields on each record in the target table. WinID does a best-match comparison in 4 ways: (i) Ranking in order of most matches, (ii) Ranking in order of least mismatches, (iii) Ranking using dental restorations only, and (iv) Ranking based on physical descriptors. To access the comparison window, a record of any ranking on one of the comparison tables is selected. A new window appears. The comparison window shows the key record as compared with the selected target record. Scroll bars enable the user to go down or up the target records list to display different comparisons.

Table 5.4: Restorative patterns

None	*One surface*	*Two surface*	*Three surface*	*Four surface*	*Five surface*	*Other*
		MO	MOD			
		MD	MOF			
	M	MF	MOL			
	O	ML	MDF	MODF		
U	D	OD	MDL	MODL		C
V	F	OF	MFL	MOFL	MODEL	X
	L	OL	ODF	MDFL		J
		DF	ODL	ODFL		
		DL	OFL			
		FL	DFL			

DIGITAL PICTURES

Progression to Possible Match

- A digital picture is not like conventional photos that have continuous tonal qualities. If one looks at a snapshot with a microscope, the higher magnifications show a smooth blend from each color to the next adjoining color. A digital picture is not made this way. A pixel (short for picture element) is the digital building block seen at higher magnifications. It is a tiny square of assigned color. Numerous pixels per square inch are needed to make a photo-quality computer print. The DPI, or dots per inch, capability of the digital computer printer corresponds to the camera or scanner's PPI, or pixels per inch, and is considered the machine's highest possible resolution setting. This is expressed with 2 numbers, which denote the width and height of the best image resolution (e.g. 1020 × 720 dpi for a certain brand of printer; ppi is substituted for digital cameras). A photo-quality digital print is considered to be 300 × 300 dpi. This hypothetical camera or printer's image capability is determined by dividing the former by the latter numbers (1020 ÷ 300, 720 ÷ 300). The result shows the largest photo-quality sized computer print of 300 dpi is 3 inches × 2 inches. Printing this image at much larger dimensions creates the jaggedy edging, which are individual pixels (pixellation). The lack of continuous color tones becomes obvious at 8 × 11 inch print size. It is necessary to use a desktop computer that can exceed the minimum equipment requirements for imaging applications (such as Adobe Photoshop 5 [Adobe Systems, Seattle, WA]) and the file sizes (between 10 and 20 megabytes for a high-resolution image) produced by these special cameras and scanners. The random access memory (RAM) in the computer should be 3 times the average image size worked on. Image applications such as Photoshop need a lot of RAM to operate reasonably fast.

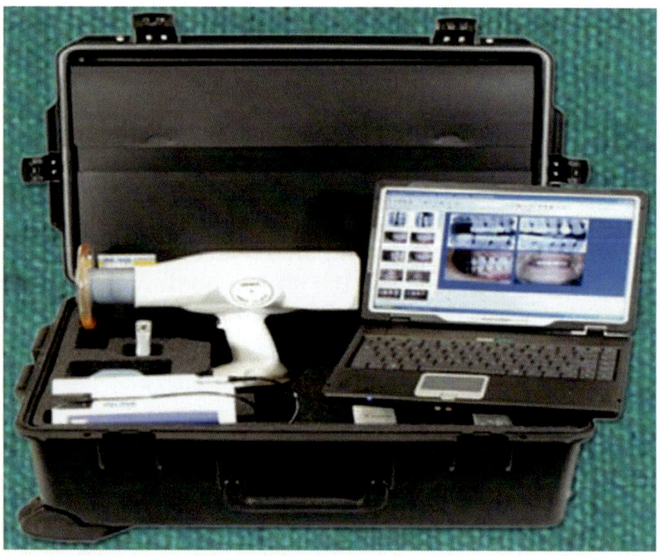

Fig. 5.2

- The radiographic determination of dental status in postmortem remains is the foundation of dental identification. This graphic representation of dental restorations, osseous landmarks, and root canal therapy is compared with records and radiographs obtained from family and personal records. This comparison searches for common points of anatomy and dental treatment that contain the same two-dimensional shapes in the Q and K evidence.
- The radiographs taken of the postmortem remains should be of the same type and similar angular orientation as the antemortem films to aid in the comparison process. Conventional radiographs can be digitized easily using a film scanner, or a digital photograph can be taken with the films mounted on a light box. Digital radiography is an excellent means of recording postmortem images.
- Computer-generated methods produce accurate and reproducible overlays when used by investigators familiar with the techniques. The following is an outline of these techniques using Adobe Photoshop 5.0. Earlier versions of Photoshop can be used, although some of the advanced features may not be available for those who wish to edit their images beyond what is described here. Photoshop 6.0 has been released and is an excellent tool for overlay fabrication. The interface (screen appearance) for Photoshop 6.0 is slightly different from the 5.0 version, although the reader should have no difficulty in this regard. Similarly, the following methods are described using a PC Windows platform; Mac users should be able to follow along without difficulty.
- The techniques described result in the production of a compound overlay. The compound overlay is similar to the traditional overlay except there is an additional layer that includes the images of the biting surfaces of the teeth within the hollow volume outlines.

CHAPTER 6

Age and Sex

- Estimation of age at death and determination of sex of the victim or remains are important guides that help in the process of identification. Teeth are among the most reliable tools in the process of identification of age, especially in the first and second decades. The stages of development can be considered as one of the most dependable indicators in assessing the age of the victim. Forensic odontology has been helpful in computing the age from the available records. It is being used in forensic archeology also, to determine the age of the individual in question.
- Development stages of dentition and craniofacial skeleton are well-established. Any disturbance during this period produces changes in these tissues and serve as life long permanent record. Even after the complete development of dentition and craniofacial skeleton certain physical, chemical and biological changes take which aid in the age estimation.
- Age of an individual is the sign of maturity which may be divided into:
  - Chronologic age
  - Anatomical age [skeletal/radiological age]
  - Dental age
  - Sexual age
  - Mental age
- Historically age assessment using teeth was first published by Edwin Saunders in 1837, who claimed that teeth provided the most reliable guide to age compared to age estimation from height which was a standard method used during that time.
- Various methods are utilized for determination of age from dentition which includes:
  - Visual or clinical method
  - Radiographic examination
  - Histological and biochemical methods
- Amongst the various methods used to estimate the age of an individual "dental age" provides "more accurate" indications during first 18 to 20 years of life. But both dentition and bone development are affected by genetic, environmental, nutritional, endocrinal factors. So chronological age doesn't coincide with skeletal or dental age.

MEDICOLEGAL IMPORTANCE OF AGE

- *Criminal responsibility:* Any act which is done by a child under the age of 7 years is not an offence (Sec 82, IPC). A child between 7 and 12 years is presumed to be capable of committing an offence. A child under the age of 12 years can't give valid consent to suffer any harm which may occur from an act done in good faith and for its benefit (Sec 89, IPC).
- *Judicial punishment:* According to the Juvenile Justice Act, 1986, " Juvenile" means a boy below 16 years and a girl below 18 years. When a juvenile commits an offence the court may direct that such person may be confined to juvenile home. No delinquent juvenile shall be sentenced to death or imprisonment.
- *Rape:* Sexual intercourse by a man with a girl under 15 years even if she is his own wife or any other girl under 16 years even with her consent is an offence (Sec 375, IPC).
- *Kidnapping:* Kidnapping a minor from lawful guardianship if the age of the boy is under 16 and that of the girl is under 18 years is an offence (Sec 361, IPC).
- *Employment:* A child below 14 years can not be employed to work in any factory or mine or in other hazardous employment.
- *Attainment of majority:* A person attains majority on the completion of 18 years and if he/she is under the guardianship of court of wards he/she attains majority on completion of 21 years (sec 3, Ind. Majority Act, 1875).
- *Marriage:* A girl under 18 years and a boy under 21 years cannot contract marriage (Child Marriage Restraint Act, 1978).
- Because of these medicolegal importance of age a person may be referred to Forensic Odontologist to

estimate the age of an individual or he may be called to estimate the age of an unknown body or remains.

Factors Used for the Age Determination using Dentition

Harvey lists the following factors as those which may aid in the dental age estimation. They are:

- Appearance of tooth germs
- Earliest detectable trace of mineralization
- Degree of completion of the unerupted tooth
- Rate of formation of enamel and formation of the neonatal line
- Clinical eruption
- Degree of completion of roots of erupted teeth
- Degree of resorption of deciduous teeth
- Attrition of the crown
- Formation of physiologic secondary dentin
- Formation of cementum
- Transparency of root dentine
- Gingival recession
- Root surface resorption
- Discoloration and staining of teeth
- Changes in the chemical composition of the teeth
- Influence of disease or malnutrition on tooth eruption
- Influence of sex on tooth eruption

Classification

Methods of Age Estimation in Forensic Dentistry

Table 6.1: Methods of age estimation

Using Dentition	*Using craniofacial skeleton*		
Natal & Neonatal period	In children (upto 14 years)	In young adults (14-20 yrs)	In adults

- Age estimation in children and young adults : Determination of age during the development of dentition can be obtained with an accuracy of "plus or minus one year" and during the early part of this period, microscopic examination of teeth may provide the age with an accuracy of "plus or minus few days". Prenatal, natal and neonatal period: Histological methods are used to assess the stage of tooth development during the premineralization period.
- Mineralization of deciduous dentition commences from two to four months in utero (20-28 months in utero). Some of the histological methods can detect early mineralization 12 weeks before being detectable in the radiographs.
- One of the earliest studies in this regard was done by Kraus and Jordan who have provided data showing various stages of premineralization and early mineralization of various deciduous teeth and first permanent molar during intrauterine development.

WEIGHT OF THE DEVELOPING DENTITION

Method of Stack

- Stack has provided a regression line of weight of growing dental tissues against the age. By weighing the teeth specimen, age of unknown can be obtained from 5 months in utero to post natal age till 7 months.

Table 6.2: Prenatal and postnatal weight of teeth

Prenatal age (weeks)	Sum of tooth weights (to nearest 5 mg)
28	60
40	460
Postnatal age (weeks)	Sum of tooth weights (to nearest 10 mg)
2	530
30	1840

- **Incremental lines of Retzius** are caused by variation in the rhythmic mineralization of enamel prisms. This rhythmic patterns may be altered by various external factors such as metabolic disturbances so that the lines may appear closer or the rest periods may be prolonged.

Neonatal Line

- Neonatal lines are present in both enamel and dentine of deciduous teeth and permanent first molars which indicate the development during the transitional period between intrauterine and extrauterine environments. So the neonatal line can be used to assess the amount of pre and post natal enamel formation.
- In the dentine incremental lines of von Ebner and contour lines of owen are present. These lines described above are used to estimate age of the neonate of fetus at death.
- Miles determined age at death by measuring the thickness of enamel and dentine from the neonatal line and divided it by appropriate daily rate of formation.
- Schour and Hoffman measured the rate of apposition of enamel and dentine as 16 mm/day.
- Teivens et al have analyzed cases of sudden infant death syndrome (SIDS) with respect to incremental lines, which may help to conclude that there is a good agreement between the enamel changes and antemortem history and other known circumstances.
- Certain drugs such as tetracycline, elements such as lead, strontium and fluoride produce characteristic incremental lines, which may help to determine the age at death.

- Sometimes these incremental patterns may also be used to match those teeth which are separated from the jaws of an individual (Cameron and sims).

Age Estimation of Children (upto 14 years)

- Odontological age estimation of children upto 14 years depends on the eruption of teeth which can be either visual or through radiographic methods.
- There are numerous studies in this subject which are conducted on different populations. Data derived from these studies are given in the form of charts based on eruption of deciduous teeth, shedding of deciduous teeth and eruption of permanent teeth. Radiographical evidence of formation of crowns and root completion have been utilized for the same purpose.
- Since we know that there are various systemic and local factors influence development of dentition it is always important to mention the average age and an expected range for a particular stage of development.
- Before discussing some of the popular methods of age estimation in children it is important to know the types of tooth eruption.

  Alveolar eruption: Alveolar eruption is related to the skeletal observation and based on whether the tooth has pierced the gingiva.

  Clinical eruption: Clinical eruption means that the tooth has pierced the gingiva and is proceeding to occlusal contact. This is again divided into three phases.
  - The tip of the cusp penetrating the gingiva
  - Emergence of the crown without reaching the occlusal plane.
  - Occlusal surfaces in contact with the antagonist

Studies

Schour and Massler Chart

- In 1941, Schour and Massler's (development of the human dentition chart) was published which is periodically updated by ADA.
- The drawings show developing dentition during various age periods which are of life size and can be used to compare with radiographs or individual tooth. This chart doesn't differentiate between males and females.

Gustafson's Chart

Gustafson's chart of dental development used four stages of tooth development namely.
- Starting of mineralization.
- Crown completion
- Eruption
- Root completion.

His chart doesn't have different data for males and females.

Moores et al Study

Moores et al have used a chart for the age estimation using 14 stages of mineralization. This can be done by using a panoramic or lateral oblique projections. The results are expressed as the mean age of attainment for each 14 stages for the developing tooth studied (+/– 2 SD). Using this chart, age from 6 months to 12 years in males and females can be estimated.

Estimation of Age in Adults (Above 20 Years)

- After the development of dentition, it becomes difficult to estimate age using teeth, Most of the methods used in adults use various regressive changes of hard and soft tissues of the teeth.
- Compared with age estimation in children using development of dentition, age estimation with the use of teeth is less accurate.

SEX

Influence of Sex on Dental Development

- Differences in the crown formation stages between the sexes are minimal but during root formation females are ahead of males. Greatest difference occurs in mandibular canine in which females are ahead upto 11 months compared with males.
- Sex difference is maximum in the mandibular dentition.
- Gleiser and Hint have derived a formula to find equivalent age for attainment of landmarks stated in Moores chart.
- Female age = 0.95 (Male age)
- Eruption of teeth is earlier in warmer countries compared with colder countries.
- Usually alveolar eruption is used as a method to determine dental age but not clinical eruption because it is less variable.

Age Estimation in Young Adults (14-20 years)

- During the period of 14-20 years, third molar can be used for estimation of age.
- Van Heerden developed a five stage system measuring the mesial root of the developing mandibular third molars. He used panoramic radiographs for this study. It was found that there was no significant difference between males and females.

Table 6.3: Stages of development of mandibular third molars

	Length (mm)	*Age* (yrs)
Stage 1 : Crown complete, radiographic evidence of root formation	3.5-5.3	16.8-16.9
Stage 2 : Root length >1/3 < 1/2	7-8.6	17.5
Stage 3 : Root length >2/3 but not complete	10-12.9	17.8-17.9
Stage 4 : Root fully formed with open apex	12-15.4	18.4-18.5
Stage 5 : Apex closed		

- Kullman et al 1995 have described a method for age estimation using mandibular third molars in which formed part of root was digitized but the precision of the age estimation was slightly inferior in this method compared with the standard method.
- In a related study kullman found that there was an overestimation of 1-1.5 years when subjective stage of root development and metric measurement of formed mandibular third molars in Swedish adolescents and concluded that age from the hand wrist radiograph is more accurate compared with the one used with mandibular third molars.

Gustafson's Method

One of the initial but still popular method was suggested by Gustafson, who used six dental changes connected with aging namely
- Attrition
- Apical migration of periodontal ligament
- Deposition of secondary dentine
- Cemental apposition
- Root resorption and
- Transparency of the root dentine
- He drew a graph of tooth points plotted against age and constructed the regression line. Gustafson claimed that the average error with his method was 3.6 years.

Johanson's Modifications

Johanson et al 1911 method to give less accurate results and modified Gustafson's method by multiple regression analysis and proposed a more accurate formula for age estimation with a standard error of 5.16 years.

Maples Findings

- Maples found that amongst six factors used in Gustafson's method root transparency was the most reliable one followed by deposition of secondary dentine, formation, attrition, migration of periodontal ligament, cemental apposition and root resorption.

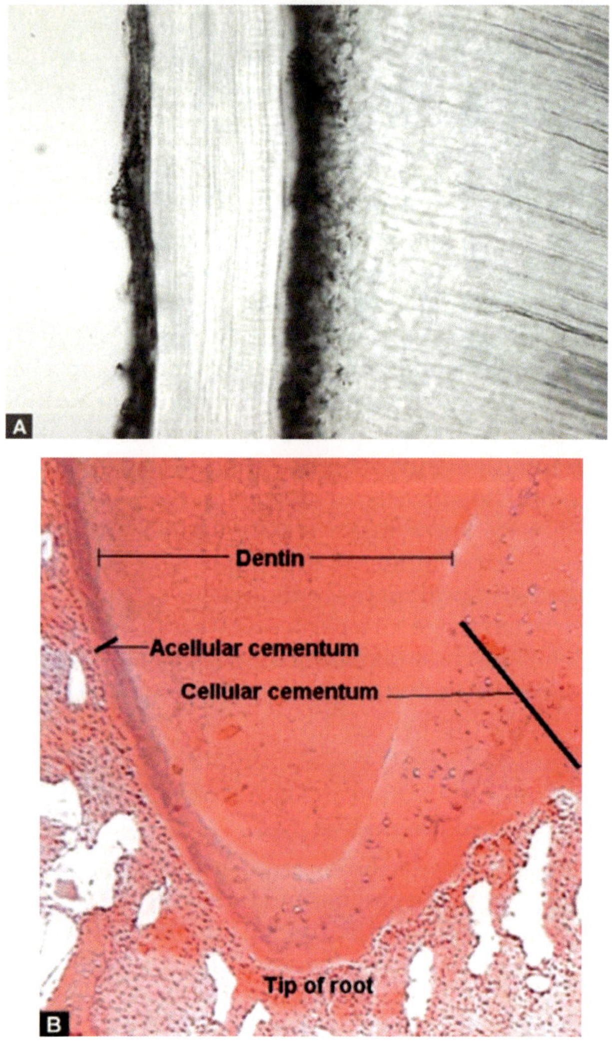

Figs 6.1A and B

- Multiple factors have always given more accurate results as compared with single factor. Some of the researchers have used individual factors for the age estimation.

Attrition

Different types of scoring methods are used by different researcher to estimate age in adults using attrition of the teeth but all of them agree that it is not a reliable index when it is used alone as it is affected by food habits, parafunctional habits, missing opposing tooth, etc.

Dentinal Root Translucency

Apical zone of translucent dentine may be used as a sole indicator of age because:
- It is less influenced by pathologic process and environmental factors.

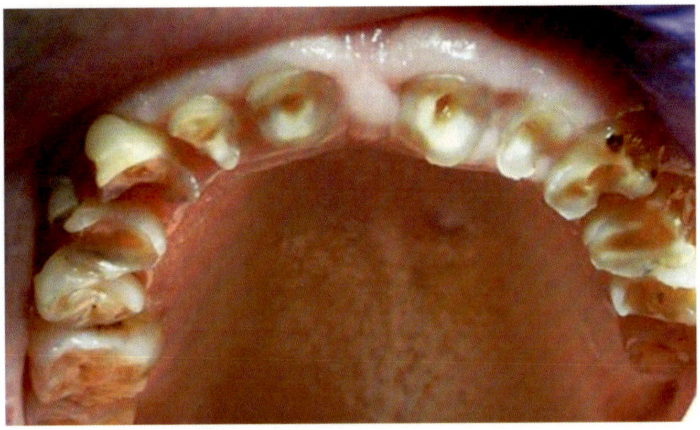

Fig. 6.2

- It shows a symmetric distribution, teeth in the left and right sides of the jaw.
- The extent of translucent zone showed little variation from one type of tooth to another.

Cause of Translucency

- Fatty degeneration of the organic substances in the dentine. Increased intratubular mineralization.
- Certain formulas are used to determine age from root dentine translucency showed high correlation with age from 0.68-0.86.
- Bang and Ramm demonstrated that the accuracy of aging with this method was 4.7 years in 58% of cases and 10 years in 79% of cases.
- In one study, it was proved that non-vital teeth have more apical translucency compared to vital tooth and slightly larger area of translucency was seen in males.

Deposition of Secondary Dentine

Size of the pulp chamber indicates the amount of secondary dentine formation. Moore used pulp diameter to crown diameter ratio for calculating age. Kvall Sl et al have used pulp/root length, pulp/tooth length and pulp/root width using periapical radiographs to estimate age by secondary dentine formation. But both the studies did not show accurate age.

Cemental Annulation Method

Cementum is continuously depsoited at the root end and seen as incremental lines. Many researchers have used cemental annulations to determine age of adults. At present there is controversy using this method because different studies show vast discrepancies in the results.

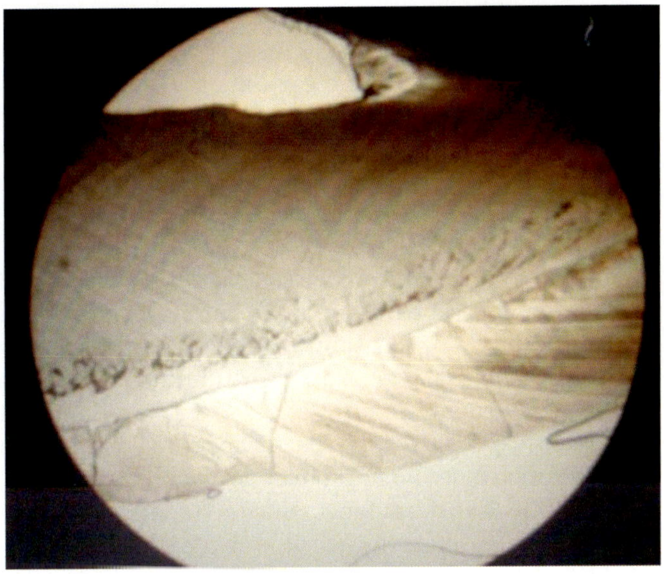

Fig. 6.3

Fluorescence from Dentine and Cementum

An interesting method using intensity of fluorescence from dentine and cementum was described by Kvaal S et al, 1995 states that who have found that there was a strong correlation between age, deepening of color of the tooth and increase in the intensity of fluorescence. It has been proposed that color changes in the dentine and cementum are caused by infusion of decomposition products from erythrocytes.

Racemization of Aspartic Acid

- A promising method is emerging as an accurate indicator of adult age using tooth is known as "racemization of aspartic acid method".
  Racemization of amino acids is an irreversible first order reaction which is relatively rapid in the living tissues that have a slow metabolic rate such as lens and tooth.
- Aspartic acid shows a high racemization rate and provides useful information about the changes occuring in the tissues over time. As the age advances there is an increase in the aspartic acid from L aspartic acid or in other words there is an increase in the D/L ratio.
- Even though, enamel, dentine and cementum are used for this techique dentine and cementum can give precise estimation of age of an individual (SD +/- 1.6-1.9).
- Due to the action of physical agents and putrification of soft tissue, the remains become skeletonized leaving

bones and teeth, Bones can be used to determine age, sex and race of the remains.

- Presence of long bone cartilages or remnants of ligaments would indicate that death occurred recently. Erosion, pitting, chalkiness and staining of the bones indicate that much of the protein content is lost and that the bones are not to recent death.
- Development of the bone can be either cartilagenous or membranous where the soft tissues are converted into hard osseous tissue in a central position from which the process of transformation spreads. At the eleventh prenatal week there are around 806 centres of bone growth, at birth about 450 while the adult skeleton has 206 bones. That means many ossification centres have found to produce adult bone.
- The time of appearace of ossification centers, site, size and degree of fusion with other parts of the bone can be used for age estimation upto 21 years with an error of plus or minus one year.
- Ossification centres appear earlier in females but the reverse is seen in the closure of the sutures of the skull.
- After 20 years assessment of age is based on the changes in the configuration and texture mostly public symphysis, skull and vertebrae are used.

Table 6.4: Age changes on craniofacial bones

Age	*Characters*
Neonatal	Edentulons jaws. Size of the orbits are relatively large.
Skull	
1 year	Fusion of midline symphysis of the mandible. Fusion of metapic suture. Lateral sphenoid synchondrosis.
3 years	Condylar portion of the occipital bone fuses with the squama.
5 years	Condylar portion of the occipital bone fuses with basiocciput.
18-21 years	Sphenoccipital synchondrosis
Sutures	
Age	Characters
25 years	Sagittal, Coronal, lambdoid sutures start to close.
32-35 years	The sagittal suture is first to close. Initially it closes near parietal foramina and the last portion to close is near bregma around 32-35 years.
40 years	Fusion of coronal suture
45 years	Lambdoid suture fuses.
60 years	Squamous portion of the temporal bone fuses with parietal bone.

Maxillary sutures: Manne et al have described a method of estimating age from the four maxillary sutures by seeing obliteration of the sutures and concluded that it can be used to give an age range if not the exact age. Radiographically union of the sutures may be identified by irregular radioopacity on either side of the suture.

Table 6.5: Mandibular angle of different age groups

Age	*Angle*
Infancy	160 - 175°
1 - 3 years	150 - 160°
6 - 12 years	125 - 140°
15 - 17 years	120 - 130°
18 - 21 years	90 - 125°
30 - 40 years	95 - 115°
40 years and above	Obtuse angle < infants

Table 6.6: Age changes of mandible

Area	*Infancy*	*Adult*	*Oldage*
Body	Shallow	Thick and long	Shallow
Ramus	Short & oblique forms an obtuse angle with the body	Less obtuse angle	Obtuse angle (140°)
Mental foramen	Near the alveolus	Midway between upper and lower margins	Near the alveolus
Condyle	Lower level than coronoid	Above the coronoid	Neck is bent backwards

- *Histomorphology of bone:* Histological methods to assess are based on the number of osteons per unit area.

Other Age Changes in the Skull

Texture: In young adults skull is smooth on both inner and outer surfaces. Around 40 to 45 years the surface becomes granular and rough.

Markings

- *Muscular markings:* Muscular markings start appearing around 25 years. Temporal line, nuchal line, attachment for masseter in the angle of the mandible are the areas where muscular markings are seen.
- *Pacchinian depressions:* Seen on both sides of the sagittal sutures, become marked with age.
- *Vascular markings:* Markings produced by middle meningeal artery become deeper.
- *Diploe:* After 50 years diploe become less vascularly channeled and there is increasing replacement by bone.
- Until puberty there is little sexual difference in the skulls. During this time only pelvis can be used for

determination of sex. After puberty, other bones used for determination of sex are sternum, long bones and craniofacial bones. Scapula and metacarpal bones may provide additional information.

- According to Krogman et al 1962 the degree of accuracy in sexing the adult skeleton is:

Entire skeleton	100%
Pelvis alone	95%
Skull alone	90%
Pelvis and skull	98%
Long bones alone	80%

Table 6.7: Skull traits of two sexes (Krogman/Narayan Reddy)

	Male	*Female*
General size	Large endocranial volume > 200 cc	Small lighter with thin walls
Architecuture	Rugged	Smooth
Glabella	More pronounced	Less pronounced
Orbits	Square, lower, smaller with rounded margins.	Rounded, higher, larger, sharp margins
Supraorbital ridges	Prominent	Less prominent
Forehead	Steeper and less rounded	Vertical, round and fantile
Frontonasal junction	Distinct angulation	Smoothly curved
Check bones	Heavier, laterally arched	Lighter and more pronounced
Zygomatic arch	More pronounced	Less pronounced
Frontal eminence	Small	Large
Parietal eminence	Small	Large
Occipital area	Muscle lines and protruberance marked	Less marked
Mastoid process	Medium to large round and blend	Small to medium smooth and pointed
i. Base	Sites of muscle insertion are marked	Less marked
ii. Digastric groove	Deep	Less deep
Condylar facet	Long and slender	Shorter and broad
Occipital condyles	Large	Small
Palate	Larger, broader, U-shaped	Small and parabola shaped
Fontal sinus	Well-developed	Less developed
Nasal aperture	High and narrower margins and sharp	Lower and broader
Foramina	Larger	Smaller
F. Magnum	Large and long	Small and round
External auditory meatus	Bony ridge along the upper border is prominent	Often absent
Mandible size	Larger and thicker	Smaller and thinner
Chin	Square	Rounded
Body height	Greater at symphysis	Smaller at symphysis
Ascending mus	Greater breadth	Smaller breadth
Gonial angle	Less obtuse (125°) Prominent and inverted	More obtuse. Not Prominent and inverted
Condyles	Larger	Smaller

CHAPTER

7

Teeth Variations

INTRODUCTION

- Variation of teeth has been an enduring interest to the clinical practitioner and the Forensic odontologist. No two teeth are alike. The day-to-day variation of teeth that we see is the norm. It is the odd, peculiar, and strange group of teeth to which we focus our attention here. They are called anomalies.

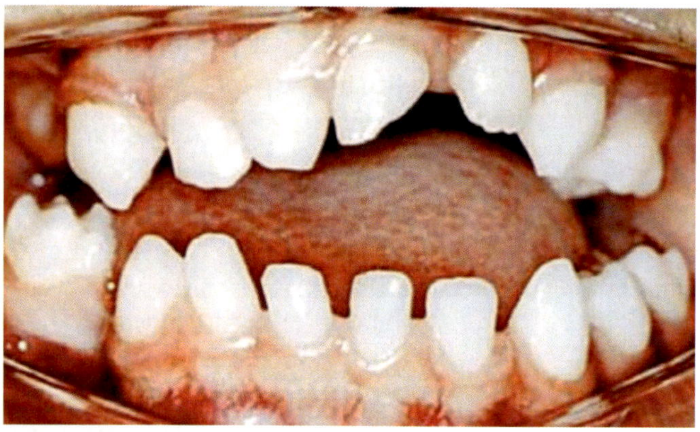

Fig. 7.1

These few facts about tooth development will assist us in understanding tooth variation:

- Teeth form from the cooperative interaction of two germ layers-ectoderm and ectomesenchyme (a neural crest derivative).
- Enamel is formed from the ectodermal components.
- Dentin, pulp, cementum, the supporting PDL, and bone are all derived from ectomesenchyme.
- Shoveling of the incisor is common amongst the Chinese, Japanese, Mongolians, and Eskimo. The Carabelli trend is most common amongst European peoples.
- Other variations, such as agenesis are useful for analysis at the biochemical and molecular level in understanding the fundamental chemistry involved in tooth formation.
- Very few heritable dental traits are truly Mendelian (although some 49 traits, many restricted to single families, are recognized). Most dental variations are polygenic, that is controlled by several genes. With these, we often speak of the degree of expression or penetrance.

DISTURBANCES IN SIZE

- Microdontia means teeth that are smaller than normal. Generalized microdontia is a rare condition associated with uncommon conditions such as pituitary dwarfism. More often, microdontia is limited to just one or two teeth. "Peg-shaped" upper lateral incisors and small third molars are seen regularly by the practicing dentist. Peg-shaped incisors tend to be familial. Occasionally, an upper lateral incisor is missing on one side, peg-shaped on the other side.

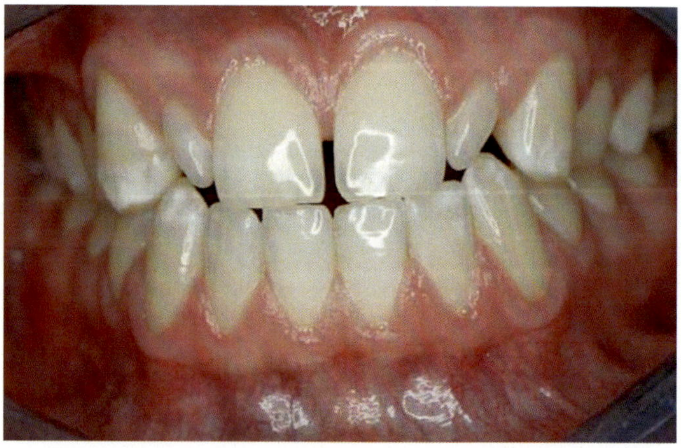

Fig. 7.2

- Macrodontia refers to teeth that are larger than normal. Generalized macrodontia is rare, seen infrequently in conditions such as pituitary gigantism. It can be localized involving just one or a few teeth. Macrodontia is much less common than microdontia.

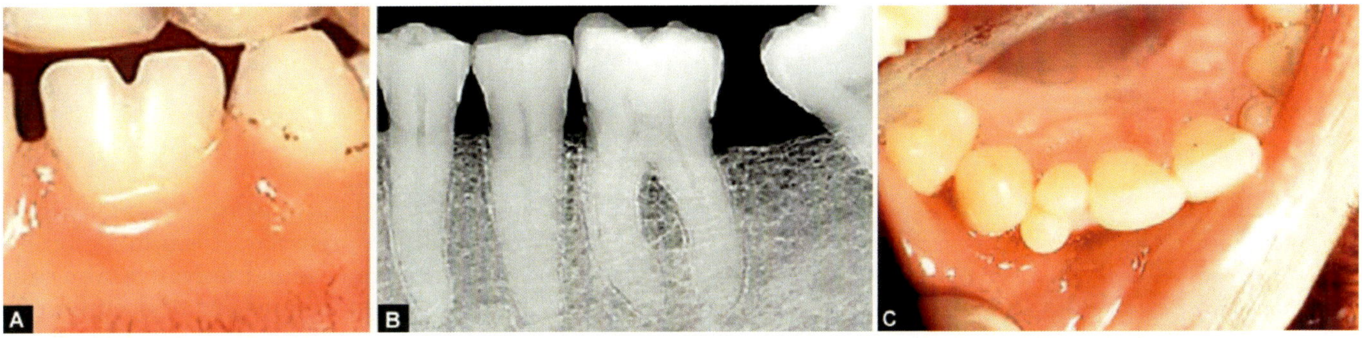

Figs 7.3A to C

DISTURBANCES IN NUMBER

- Anodontia is the congenital absense of all teeth. Edentulous means the clinical absence of teeth. Anodontia means the failure of teeth to form at all. In true (or complete) anodontia, all teeth fail to develop.
- True anodontia is an extremely rare occurrence. When this does occur, it is usually part of a more generalized disorder ectodermal dysplasia, an inherited defect of all ectodermally derived structures.
- Partial anodontia is the failure of one or more teeth to develop. It is much more common than complete anodontia. Third molars, lower second premolars, and upper lateral incisors (in that order) are the most common congenitally absent teeth. Congenital absence of a deciduous tooth is not common. When it does occur, it is most often the upper lateral incisor that is absent. When a deciduous tooth is absent, its permanent successor is usually missing also.

  Terms such as oligodontia or hypodontia are used to describe the condition of partial anodontia.
- Supernumerary teeth are 'extra' teeth. Most (90%) occur in the maxilla. Their presence in the deciduous dentition is quite rare. The most common of all supernumerary teeth is the mesiodens which is a supernumerary that forms in the midline between and lingual to the roots of the maxillary central incisors. Most supernumerary teeth do not erupt; they often are unknown until detected on X-ray films. Fourth molars, themselves a rare occurrence are infrequently called 'paramolars' or 'distomolars'. Supernumerary teeth occur less often than do missing teeth.

DISTURBANCES IN ERUPTION

- Premature eruption of all of the teeth, either deciduous or permanent, may suggest an underlying endocrine dysfunction such as hyperthyroidism. A natal tooth seen at birth may be an aberrant 'tooth' nodule, or it may actually be a deciduous incisor that has erupted early. The etiology is unknown.
- Delayed eruption can be due to local or systemic factors. For one or a few teeth, surgical exposure and if needed—orthodontic guidance can bring the tooth into its proper place. X-ray films are useful in evaluating early or late eruption of teeth.
- Impacted teeth are those that have failed to erupt and remain buried in the alveolar bone. Usually, some barrier to eruption will be seen on the X-ray film. A seldom used term for unerupted teeth is embedded teeth. The third molars and maxillary canine are the most frequently impacted teeth, followed by premolars and supernumerary teeth.
- Ectopic eruption is another type of eruption disturbance; this occurs when a tooth cannot complete its eruption because it is blocked by an adjacent tooth or by a misplaced orthodontic band-usually on a first molar tooth.
- An iatrogenic disease or condition is one that is 'doctor - caused'. If a second molar is inadvertently impacted by a poorly placed molar band it is an iatrogenic condition.
- Dilaceration is a severe bend in the long axis of the tooth. The bend is located at the junction between the crown and the root. The bend can be as much as 90 degrees. Dilaceration usually results from trauma to the unfinished tooth when development is in progress. Such a tooth in the old literature is sometimes called a 'hawk billed tooth'.
- Flexion is a deviation or bend restricted just to the root portion of the tooth. Usually the bend is less than 90 degrees. It may be a result of trauma to the developing tooth. Carefully contrast and compare the definitions for flexion and dilaceration.
- Taurodontism literally means 'bull-like teeth'. Taurodont teeth are usually molars. They have an abnormally long pulpal chamber and shortened roots.

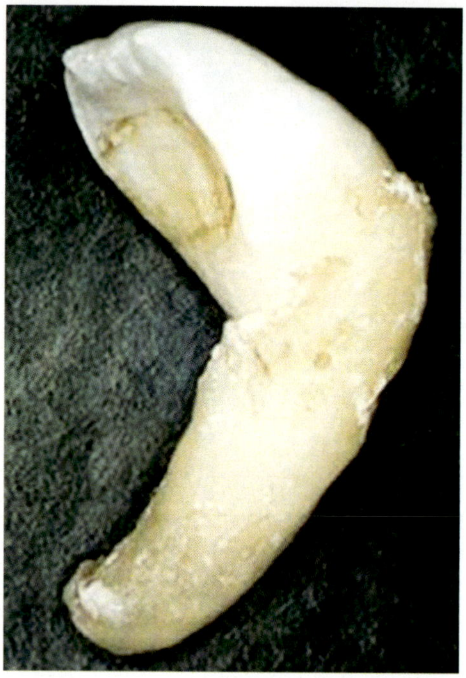

Fig. 7.4

The pulp chamber has no constriction near the CEJ as do normal teeth. Clinically, these teeth appear normal. No treatment of the condition is necessary apart from due prudence when doing root canal therapy.

- Dens in dente literally means 'tooth within a tooth'. It is a uncommon developmental abnormality that primarily affects maxillary lateral incisors. It is in fact a deeply invaginated lingual pit with an important clinical implications: These are very susceptible to caries and they ought to be restored promptly. Left unattended, these teeth tend to decay very rapidly. This condition is also called dens invaginatus.
- Supernumerary cusps, or are often called, extra cusps are occasionally found on teeth.
- The most common one is the Carabelli Cusp which is found on the mesiolingual aspect (on the mesiolingual cusp) of maxillary first molars and maxillary second deciduous molars.
- This occlusal landmark can appear with varying degrees of intensity either as a cusp of pit. These condition are known collectively as the Carabelli trait. It is frequently a site of early dental caries.
- A talon cusp is an extra cusp that resembles an eagle's talon (a talon is the claw of a bird of prey). A talon cusp appears as a projection from the cingulum of incisor teeth. These can interfere with occlusion; however, grinding them down is a hazardous endeavor. Talon cusps often contain a prominent pulp horn which is very susceptible to exposure in the younger patient.
- Very rarely, a similar projection of enamel can occur on the occlusal surface of the premolar teeth. It forms a tubercle called a 'dens evaginatus'. Dens evaginitus can also contain a pulp horn.
- One other variation of the upper first premolar is the 'Uto-Aztecan' upper premolar. It is a bulge on the buccal cusp that is only found in Native American Indians, with highest frequencies of occurence in Arizona.
- Peg-shaped lateral incisor have root variation. teeth exhibit a variation in the number of roots. Most root variation is in the distal third of the root. Sometimes roots can be blunted or shortened. It tends to occur without apparent cause. Root resorption and root blunting can be unfortunate consequence of orthodontic treatment with fixed appliances.
- Upper first premolars usually have two roots; however, one root is occasionally found in these teeth. More rarely there are three roots.
- Lower permanent canines on occasion have a bifurcation near the apex resulting in two short roots.
- Sometimes lower first permanent molars have three roots. It is the mesial molar root that is bifurcated. It is just a variation. Three rooted lower first molars are found in greater frequency amongst North American Indian with origins in Asia.
- In upper third molars, and on occasion with fused roots, second molars, the roots can be fused together. This is a variation, not a pathological condition.
- Shovel-shaped incisor display enhanced marginal ridges and present with a distinctive shovel-shaped appearance on the lingual aspect.
- Fusion is the union of two teeth by dentin and enamel. The pulp chambers are often shared, however, they can be separate. This condition can be differentiated from gemination by counting the teeth. The diagnosis can be confirmed, if there is a reduction in the number of teeth that are present in the dental arch. Some refer to fusion as 'syndontism'.
- Gemination is the development of two crowns from a single tooth germ. It is an incomplete twinning of the gooth germ. In gemination, there is a shared pulp and root. Some refer to gemination as 'schizodontism'.
- Concrescence is the joining of tooth roots by cementum. A missed diagnosis can be serious complication during an attempted extraction.
- A related occurrence is hypercementosis. It is a consequence of excessive cementum deposition. It occurs in older people often when there are greatly increased or decreased occlusal forces.

DISTURBANCES IN FORMATION

- Enamel pearls (enamelomas) are small nodules of enamel found on the root of the tooth close to or at the cemento-enamel junction. They are found most often at the bifurcation or trifurcation of molars. They do appear radiographically. While they can be a problem in periodontal disease, they should usually be left alone. Their attempted removal can do more harm than good.
- Hutchinson's incisors or mulberry molars are developmental anomalies that result from congenital syphilis. Clinically, the incisor teeth are, on occasion called 'screwdriver teeth' due to their distinctive shape.
- Winged incisor are not a disturbance of development, but rather a special case of rotation of the upper central incisors. It is usually described as a distinctive bilateral rotation to the mesial which is particularly common amongst Native American Indians.
- Enamel hypoplasia can be localized or generalized. Localized enamel hypoplasia is a visible defect that is important in archaeology as an indicator of severe sickness or nutritional deprivation. When the insult during tooth formation is brief in duration, it can be detected histologically in the enamel as a Wilson's line.

CHAPTER 8

Bitemarks

INTRODUCTION

- Bitemark injuries McDonald et al (1981) States that are a form of "patterned injury" which means that the configuration is caused by a particular object. Sometimes bitemarks are called as "toolmarks".

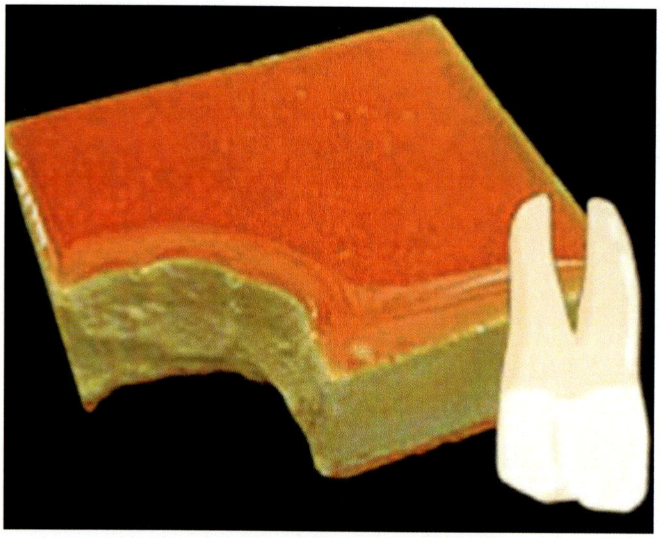

Fig. 8.1

- McDonald has defined bitemark as "a mark made by the teeth either alone or in combination with other mouth parts".
- Historically distinctive nature of tooth arrangement had legal implications. William the conqueror validated royal documents by biting into a wax seal with his characteristic dentition. Debtors from Britain when came to America to work, used to bitethe seal on the agreement pacts in lieu of a signature and became known as "indentured servants". One of the earliest investigator recognized as bitemarks analyst was Sorup, who in 1942 used transparent paper representations of a suspect's dentition to compare with life sized bitemark photograph. The first case

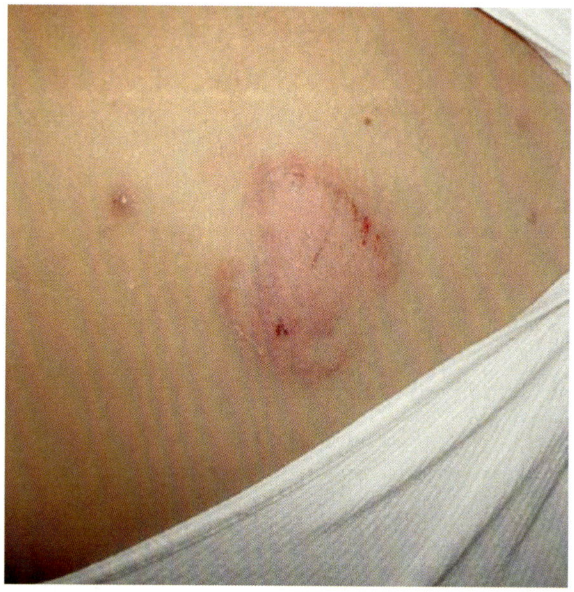

Fig. 8.2

involving a bitemark that led to a conviction sustained upon appeal was a 1972 rape case. Since then there are number of cases reported involving bitemark evidence.
- Analysis of bitemarks has improved with advanced and accurate techniques to evaluate, match and present bitemark cases. Bitemark evidence is admissible under Frye test, which deal with admissibility for scientific evidence. It has three requirements. They are:
  - The scientific principle must be recognizable.
  - The scientific principle must be sufficiently established.
  - The scientific principle must have gained acceptance in the discipline to which it belongs.

CRIMES INVOLVED IN BITEMARKS

Bitemarks may be found on living or dead individuals where the person may be victim of the crime or perpetrator of the crime. Bitemarks may also be seen in the food substance or inanimate objects at the crime scene. Bitemarks may be produced during assault of children or adults which are frequently associated with sex related crimes and child abuse.

Location: According to Vale et al arms were the most frequent sites followed by the breasts, legs, abdomen, back, face, shoulder, buttocks, female genitalia, hand, chest, neck, nose, male genitalia ear and foot.

CLASSIFICATION OF BITEMARKS

According to agents producing marks:

Humans	-	Adults
	-	Children
Animals	-	Mammals (e.g. dog)
		Reptiles (e.g. snake)
		Fish
Mechanical	-	Dentures
	-	Saw blade, etc.

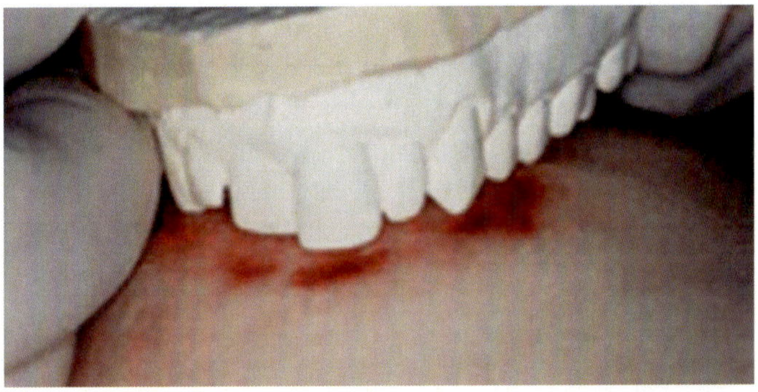

Fig. 8.3

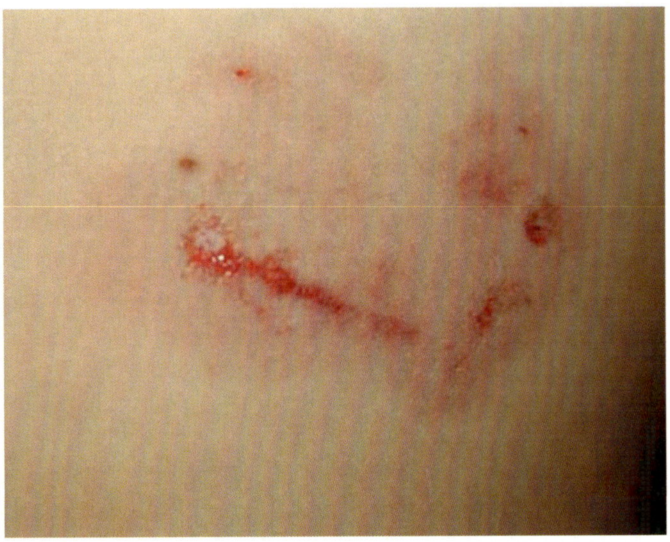

Fig. 8.4

According to the materials in which bitemarks are produced:

- Skin and body tissues
- Food substances

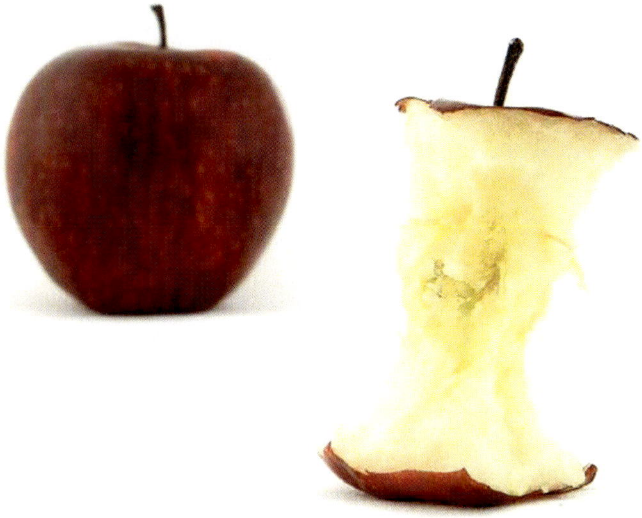

Fig. 8.5

- Other materials chewed habitually, e.g. pipe stems, pens and pencils.
- *Pressure exerted while biting:* The pressure exerted by teeth while biting is around 11 kg from the incisors and from tongue may reach upto 8 lb/square inch. Suction is a distinct form of thrust from the tongue and it may produce a negative pressure of 20 mm Hg.

TYPES OF BITEMARKS

- *Sexually oriented bites:* Sexially oriented bites appear to have been inflicted slowly and deliberately with suction applied to the tissue by tongue and lips. The resultant injury exhibits central or peripheral "suck marks" and marks of anterior teeth with good definition. The amount of distortion may indicate whether the person being bitten was active or passive when the bitemark was being inflicted.
- *Child abuse cases:* In the child abuse cases either aggressive (anger bitemarks) or sexually oriented type of bitemarks are seen.
- *Self-inflicted bitemarks:* Mostly found on the forearms of children caused by themselves. Sometimes arms may be pushed into the child's mouth to stop crying or due to intense pain children may bitethemselves because of fear. Mentally retarded and psychologically disturbed people may also inflict biteon themselves. Self-inflicted bitemarks are also seen in Lesch-Nyhan syndrome, a X-linked, recessively transmitted disease with intensitivity to pain.

FACTORS INFLUENCING THE BITEMARKS

- *Type of tissue:* In the case of skin, if it is loose or with excessive fat bites commonly produce bruising leading to poor definition. Whereas in areas of fibrous tissue or with high muscle content tend to bruise less, so that the definition of bitemark is good.
- *Age:* Infants and old individuals bruise more than other age groups.
- *Sex:* Females tend to bruise more than males. Once produced bitemarks will be evident for longer period of time in females compared to males.
- *Medical status:* People having bleeding disturbances, under anticoagulant therapy and certain skin diseases bruise more.
- *Time:* The time elapsed between actual biting and when the impression is made is vital. Depression produced in the skin due to bitemarks will recover within 10-20 minutes leaving swelling and discoloration. After death skin tends to contract, harden and decompose.
- *Histopathologic changes:* Histopathologic changes according to the age of bitemark in the skin is given below:

Table 8.1: Histopathological changes of healing of bitemarks

Time (hours)	*Predominant cells and deposits*	*Healing*	*Clinical color*
4 - 8	PMNL	-	Red/blue/purple
12	PMNL	-	-
16 - 24	Macrophages	Peripheral	Blue to black fibrosis
24 - 36	PMNL	-	-
Days			
1 - 3	Central necrosis	Green to blue	
3 +	Hemosiderin	Collagen fibers	
4	-	Capillary growth	Brown to yellow green
4 - 5	-	Lymphocytes	
10 - 14	-	Granulation tissue	Tan yello
Stage - 1	-	Scab formation	(0 to 18 hours)
Stage - 2	-	Epithelial regeneration	(30 to 70 hours)
Stage - 3	-	Subepidermal granulation	(5 - 12 days)
Stage - 4	-	Regression	(After 12 days)

Enzyme histochemistry: According to Rae Kallio, the appearance of various enzymes from the time of injury are as follows:

ATPase	:	1 hour after injury
Esterase	:	1 hour after injury
Acid phosphatase	:	4 hours after injury
Alkaline phosphatase	:	8 hours after injury

Biochemical Studies

- Biochemical study can differentiate bitecaused before and after death. There is no increase in 5HT or free histamine in postmortem wounds. But a distinct increase in these compounds indicates antemortem origin of a wound.
- *Immunological studies:* Antemortem wounds contain glycoprotein—A of erythrocytic membranes. Since marks fade rapidly, bitemarks should be examined as soon as possible.

Force exerted by the biter, number and type of teeth, presence of tongue thrust, can alter the way the teeth contact a bitten surface. TMJ problems may lead to midline shift. Marks caused in dead shows absence of bleeding into the injury and absence of inflammatory reaction surrounding the tissue injury.

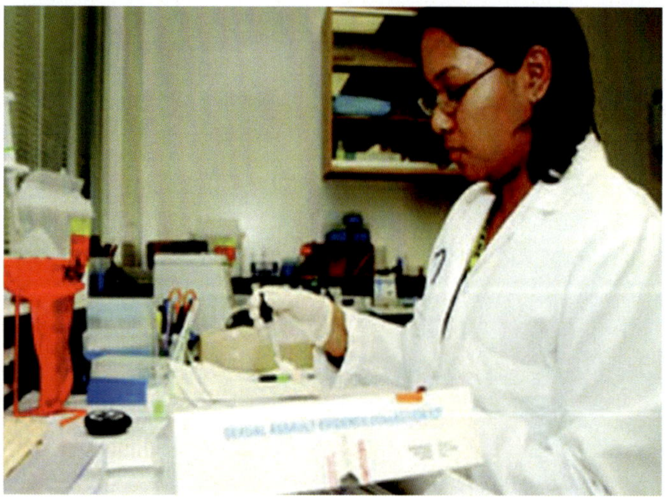

Fig. 8.6

Controversies Regarding Bitemark Evidence

Unlike finger prints there are number of factors which can alter the bitemark evidence. So there is controversy regarding the legal status of bitemark evidence. Errors in recording, comparison, analysis and interpretations of bitemarks may lead to serious consequences. There is also debate regarding the minimum constitution and composition of the bitemark required for effective evaluation. So, many attempts have been made to establish "standards" for gathering evidence and interpretation of evidence. ABFO guidelines are one of the accepted standards for bitemark analysis.

Definitions of Marks in Forensic Dentistry (Jakobsen)

Tooth mark	:	Mark left by a tooth.
Arch mark	:	Mark produced by four or five adjacent teeth in the same arch.
Bitemark	:	Tooth marks produced by antagonistic teeth.

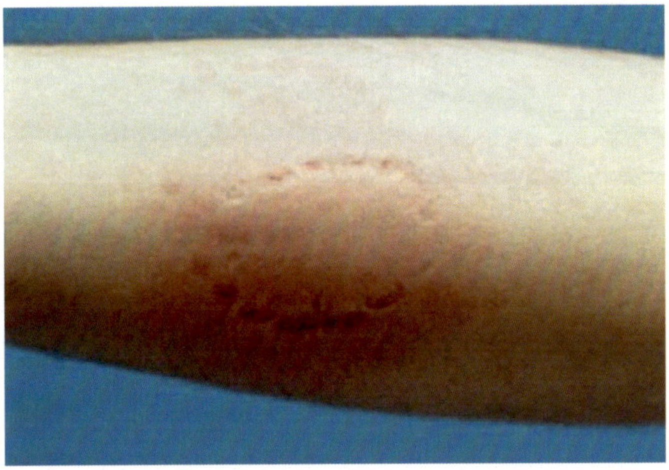

Fig. 8.7

Bitemark cases have to be dealt step by step in the following way:

- Description of bitemarks
- Collection of evidence from the victim
- Collection of evidence from the suspect
- Bitemarks comparison.

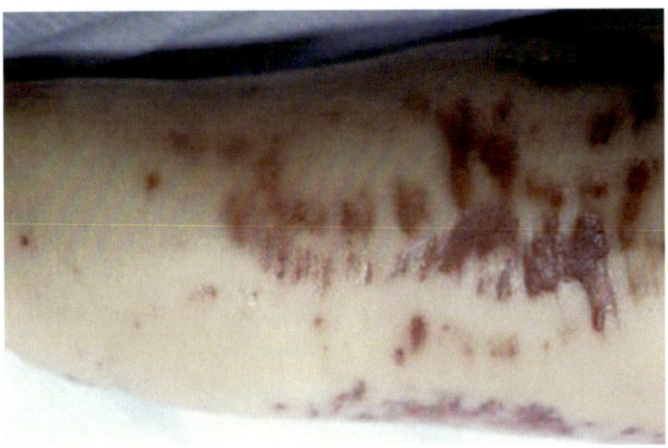

Fig. 8.8

Description of Bitemarks

Both in the living and deceased victims the following vital information should be recorded.

Demographics

Name, age, sex, race, case number, date of examination, and name of the examiners should be recorded.

Location of the Bitemark

- Describe the anatomic location, indicate the contour of the surface as flat, curved or irregular and state the tissue characters.
- Sin—fixed or mobile.
- Underlying tissue—bone, cartilage, muscle or fat.

Shape of the Bitemarks

Indicate whether it is round, ovoid, crescent or irregular in shape.

Color of the Mark, Size of the Mark

Both vertical and horizontal dimensions should be recorded in metric system.

Type of Injury

- Type of tissue injury due to bitemark may be
- Petechial hemorrhage
- Contusion
- Abrasion
- Laceration
- Incision
- Avulsion
- Artefact.

Note: The surface of the skin as smooth or indented.

Data Collection from the Victim

Bitemark evidence should be gathered from the victim after obtaining authorization from the authorities. Determine whether the bitemark has been affected by washing, contamination, embalming, decomposition, etc.

Steps in the Examination of the Victim

Photographs of the bitemarks should be made immediately.

SALIVARY SWABBING

The amount of saliva deposited with a bitemark is about 0.3 ml and distributed over a wide area of 20 cm practical points helpful in the collection of salivary swabbing are described below.

- One square centimeter piece of Rizla type of cigarette paper held in forceps is used after wetting it with fresh water or distilled water (contamination with fingers will give false positive result). The whole bitemark and the adjacent area should be swabbed. Air dry the paper by placing it on a clear microscopic slide. After drying swabs are packed and send to the laboratory. A control sample is prepared using same method as described above but without swabbing with saliva. Instead of using paper, a cotton piece can also be used for saliva swabbing.

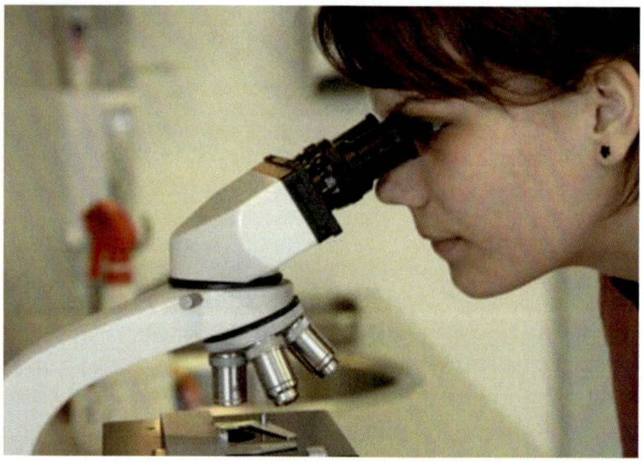

Fig. 8.9

- Saliva obtained from swabbing is used to determine the blood group antigens. Identification of the saliva is done by demonstrating it's amylase activity in hydrolyzing a starch substrate. The presence of blood group antigens can be determined by absorption-elution or absorption—inhibition group testing.
- In the case of sexual assault, oral swabs should also be taken for semen. Mouth washes (with water) can be used to obtain test sample for spermatozoa.

Impression of Bitemarks

If the bitemarks have penetrated the skin, an impression of the marks should be made. A rubber base material such as vinyl polysiloxans with dimensional stability should be used. Two methods are commonly used to make impression.

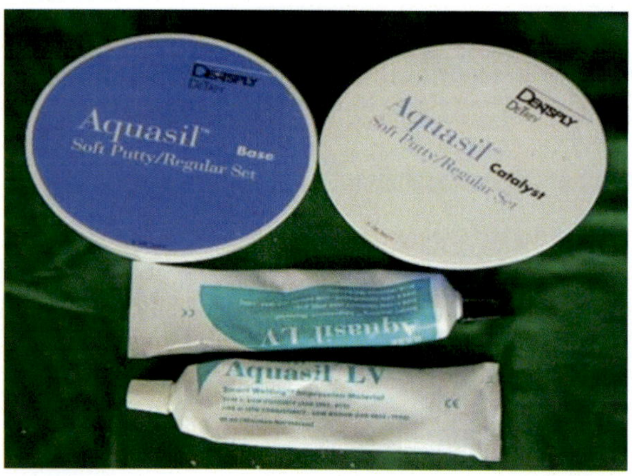

Fig. 8.10

Method I

- Cover the bitearea with 5 mm thick light bodied material.
- Place a wire gauze over the set material.
- Inject additional material over it.
- After removal of the impression indicate the direction of head with marker on the back of the impression.

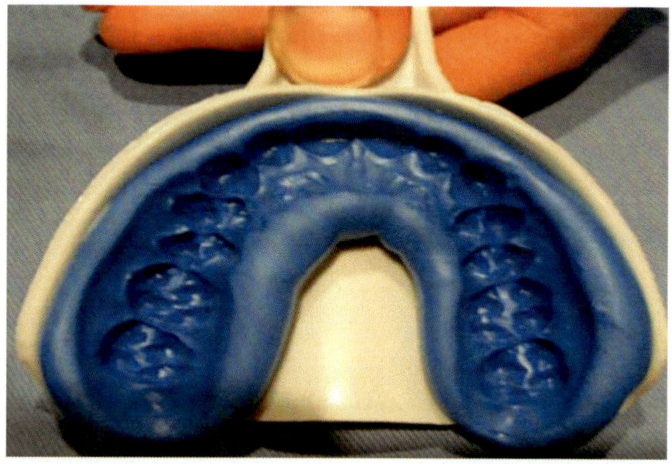

Fig. 8.11

Method II

- A special tray is constructed using cold cure or orthopedic cast material confining to the shape of anatomic part in which bitemark is present. Impression is made using rubber base material.

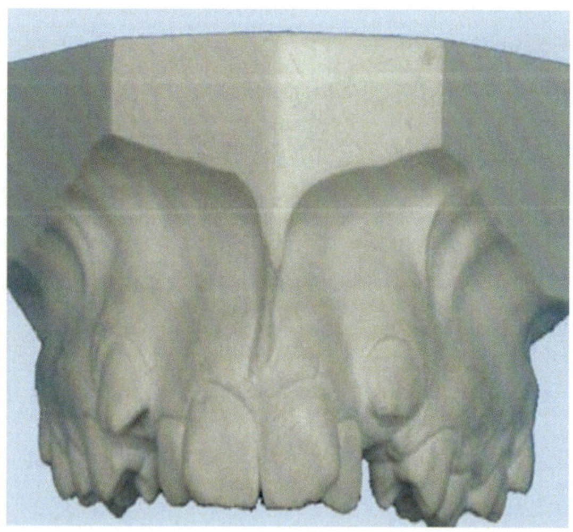

Fig. 8.12

- Master casts must be poured with type-IV stone and duplicate casts should also be made. Either visible light cure or epoxyresin clear material may be used to make stable rigid model.

Bite Print Recording

Similar to the method used to lift finger prints from crime scenes, finger print lifting tape can be used to lift the "non-perforating" bitemarks after brushing the bitemark with finger print lifting powder.

Tissue Samples

In the case of dead victims with bitemarks, bitemarks can be excised along with the underlying tissues after fixing an acrylic stent around the bitemark to avoid shrinkage of the tissue. Store the specimen in 4 percent formalin.

Examination of the Suspect

Following details should be noted from the suspect after obtaining necessary consent. History of dental treatments after or just before the bitemark has to be noted.

Photographs

Full face, profile photographs, frontal, occlusal and lateral views of the dental arches should be taken.

Examination

- TMJ status, facial asymmetry, muscle tone, maximum opening of mouth, deviation while opening and closing movements have to be recorded under extra oral examination. Tongue movements, periodontal status should be noted. Special attention should be given to the arrangement of dentition.
- C. saliva swabbing should be performed as described before.

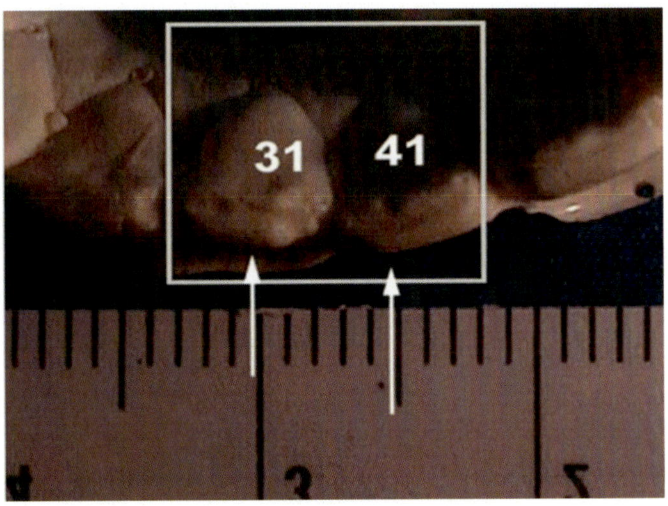

Fig. 8.13

- D. upper and lower dental models should be prepared.
- Sample bites should be made whenever possible, simulating the type of biteunder study. This may be recorded in wax sheet or in impression compound.

Evaluation of Evidence

- American Board of Forensic Odontology (ABFO) has provided a scoring system which gives scores for gross features, tooth position and intradental features for evaluating the evidence collected from bitemarks.
- While evaluating the bitemark firstly the cause of the mark has to be determined, since bitemarks may be caused by nonhumans or humans. Following two factors will help to differentiate bitemarks caused by nonhuman from human.

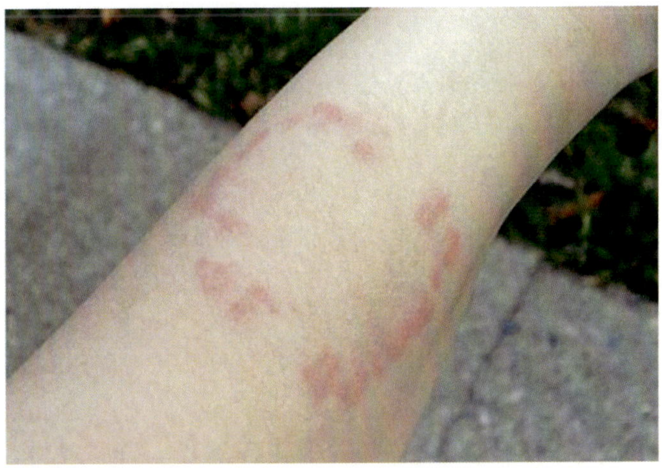

Fig. 8.14

TEETH SIZE, SHAPE AND ARRANGEMENT IN THE ANTERIOR PORTION OF THE ARCH

Human incisor teeth produce rectangular marks whereas canine teeth produce triangular marks in cross-section. Animal bites inflicted by dogs or cats puncture the skin and the cross-sectional size of the tooth is small and circular. Number of incisor teeth may be greater with animal bites and the distance between individual teeth is greater than mesiodistal width of the teeth.

Size of the Dental Arch

Width of the adult arches from canine to canine is 2.5-4 cm. Children's arches are smaller than the adults whereas dog's and cat's arches are smaller than children.

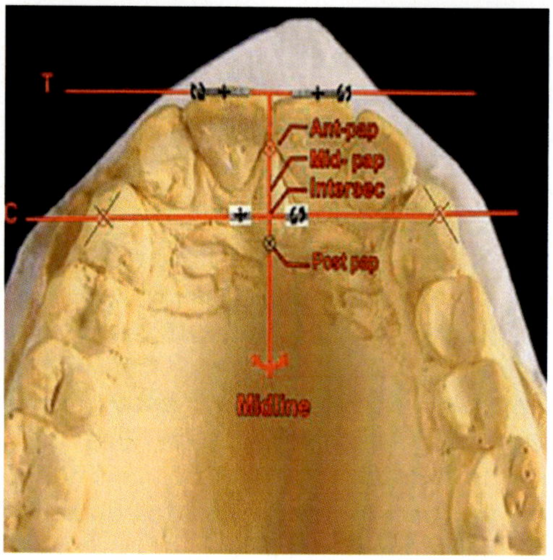

Fig. 8.15

Evaluation of the Bitemark Photographs

Attempts should be made to thoruoughly analyze the bitemarks *in vivo* and *in vitro* rather than mere superimposition of marks in the photograph over the models.

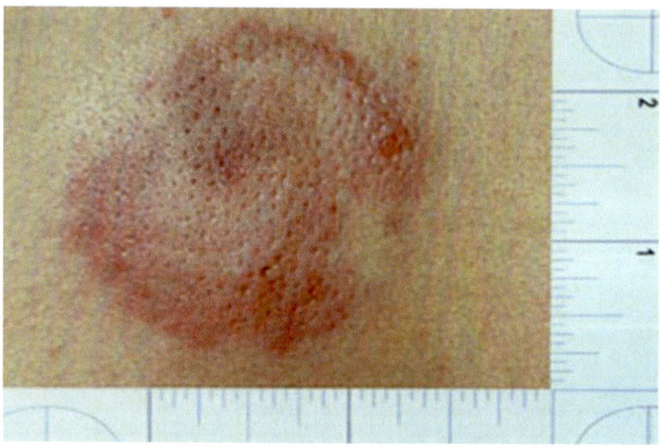

Fig. 8.16

Evaluation of the Arches

Shape of the arch should be noted as circular, ellipsolid or elongated. Central lines of upper and lower arches should be established.

Suction Marks

Some claim that the presence of suction marks in the centre of the arch marks is a sign of bitemark of human origin. But now it is considered that suction marks are caused due to injury to the blood vessels when compressed between the jaws of the biter.

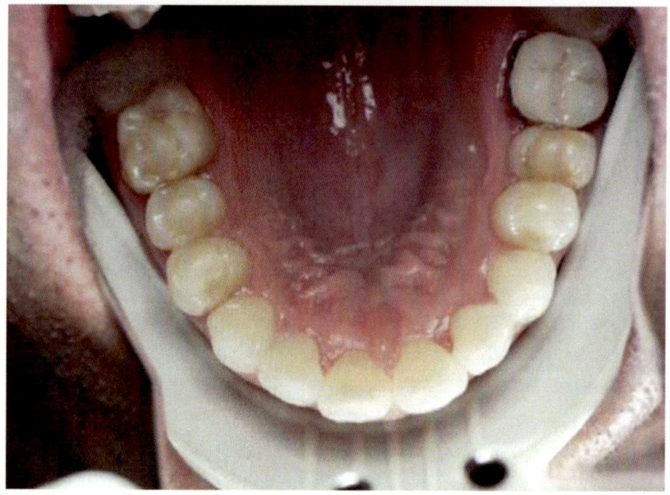

Fig. 8.17

Characteristics in the Mark

Ascertain the characteristics of individual marks within the arch. Areas of abrasion, laceration or bruising may indicate occlusal level of a particular tooth or a sharp cusp. Tooth numbers should be identified. Placement of tooth marks in the arch (labial/lingual placement) and missing teeth should be noted.

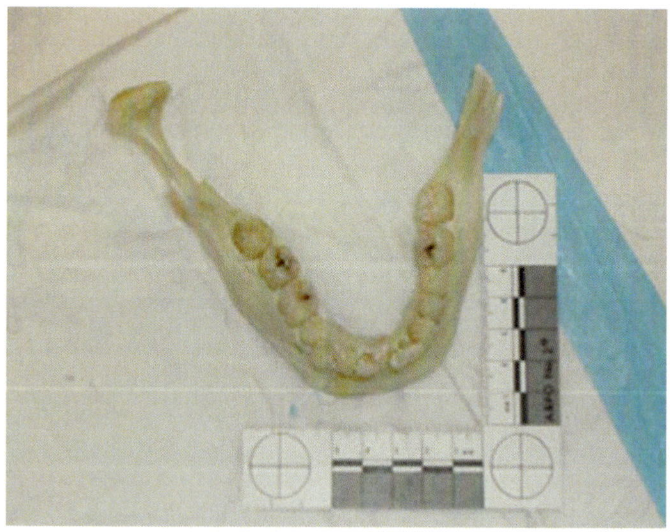

Fig. 8.18

MACDONALD'S CLASSIFICATION OF BITEMARKS

Tooth Pressure Marks

Tooth pressure marks are caused by incisal edges of the anterior teeth. They are stable and subjected to minimal distortion.

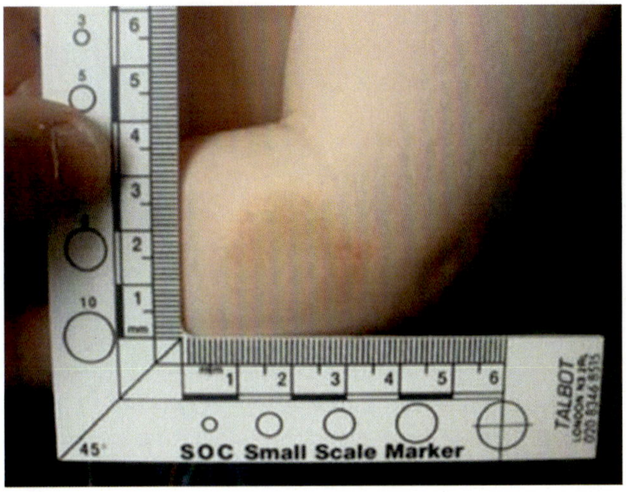

Fig. 8.19

Tongue Pressure Marks

Because of the tongue pressure, impressions of the palatal surfaces of the teeth, cingulae or palatal rugae may be produced. This causes distortion of the marks.

Tooth Scrape Marks

Scrape marks are produced because of irregularities in the teeth due to fractures, restorations, etc.

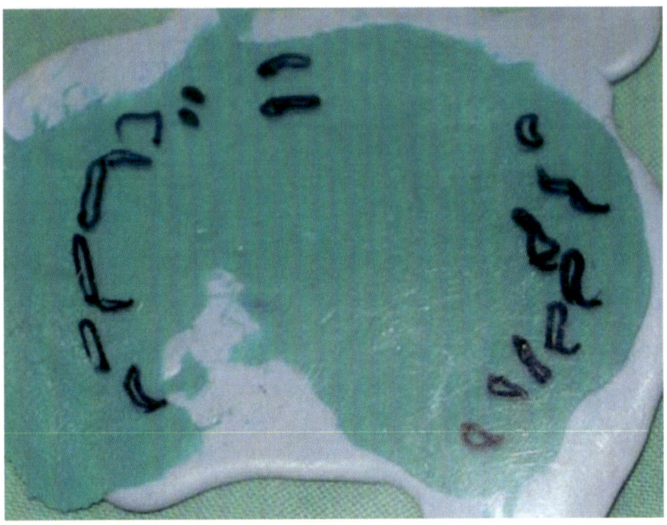

Fig. 8.20

Complex Marks

Combination of the above types of marks. According to jakobsen et al the shape of the bitemark depends on the amount of tissue taken into the mouth. For example, an ellipsoid shape may indicate that only small amount of tissue is taken inside the mouth and only anterior teeth are used to bite. On the other hand marks showing premolar teeth in both the arches are usually circular in shape.

METHOD OF ANALYSIS OF BITEMARKS

Odontometric Triangle Method

- In this objective method, a triangle is made on the tracing of bitemarks and teeth models by marking three points, two on the outer most convex point of canines and one in the centre of the upper central incisors. Three angles of the triangles are measured and compared.
- A clinico-anthropological study carried out by Manohar Singh et al by comparing bitemark width, bizygomatic and bigonial width concluded that from a given bitemark impression the facial dimensions of a person who is responsible for the mark can be determined.

Comparison Techniques

Comparison techniques can be classified as direct and indirect methods. They use life size 1:1 photographs and models of teeth. In assisted comparison method, specialized techniques such as microscopic methods, radiographs or experimental bitemarks are used.

Direct Method

Model from the suspect can be directly placed over the photograph of the bitemark to demonstrate concordant points. Videotape can be used to show slippage of teeth producing distorted images and to study dynamics of the bitemarks.

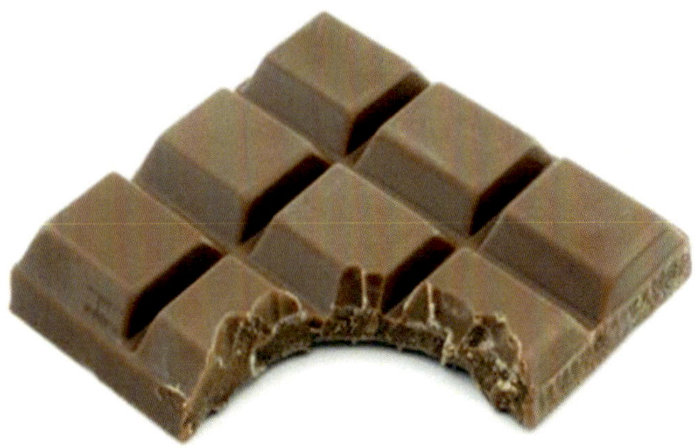

Fig. 8.21

Indirect Method

Indirect method involve preparation of transparent overlay of occlusal or incisal surfaces of the teeth which are then placed over the marks on the photographs. Over lays may be produced by tracing the occlusal surface of teeth by placing cellulose acetate paper over the model. Xeroxing the model on the transparent sheet, use of reverse negatives which preserves the anatomic details, recording bitein a wax sheet or sprinkling radiopaque powders into the teeth impression, then producing a radiograph. CT scan can be used to produce overlays of the dentition at varying depths. This is considered to be an accurate method of overlay production.

Special Methods in Bitemark Analysis

- *Vectron:* Vectron is used to measure distances between fixed points and angles.
- *Stereometric graphic analysis:* This can be used to produce contour map of the suspect's dentition.
- *Experimental marks:* Experimental bitemarks may be produced on the pig sking, bakers dough or rubber for analysis.
- *Result:* In comparing a particular bitemark, it is important to respond affirmatively, negatively or stating that the evidence is insufficient for a firm conclusion.

Bitemarks in Inanimate Objects

- In the literature bitemarks found in a variety of inanimate objects such as wooden cabinets, pipe stems, mouth pieces of musical instruments and more commonly in the food stuffs, such as cheese, chocolate, apples, chewing gums etc have been reported.

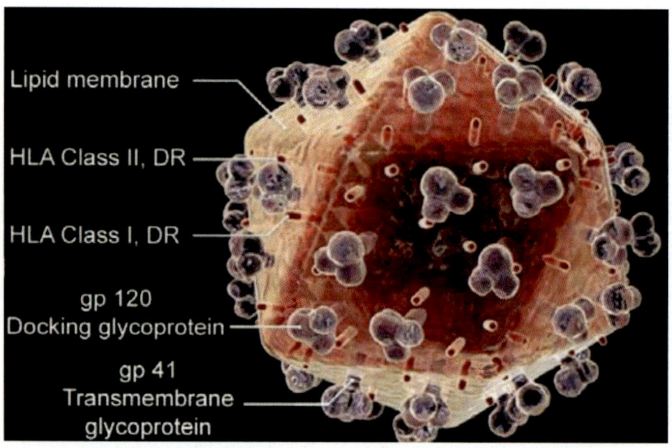

Fig. 8.22

- Terminologies such as three dimensional bite, tentative bite, complete bite, sliding biteare used to describe bitemarks in food. To overcome this confusion Webster classified them into three types.
  - *Type I:* Bites that are found in materials such as chocolate, which fracture readily with a limited depth of penetration. Bites of this type will record the most prominent incisal edges of the upper and lower anterior teeth up to a depth of 1-2 mm.
  - *Type II:* Bites in this type consist of those where a good group of the material is obtained by the teeth and then the bitten piece is removed by fracturing it from the main material, e.g. apple. This type of biteshows a record of the outline of labial aspect of upper and lower incisors and tooth scrape marks tend to record those elements of teeth which are most prominent anteriorly.
  - *Type III:* Bites of this type are produced by biting through the material such as cheese. It has an advantage that it indicates relative positions of upper and lower incisors in centric occlusion from the extensive scrape marks.

Since the bitemarks in food substances may produce exact mesiodistal dimension of teeth, records should be made as soon as possible. Saliva swabbing can be taken from the bitemark for blood group analysis.

Preservation

- Storage of the food materials with bitemark can be done by placing them in air tight bags and then in refrigerator or by using preserving solutions (made up of equal parts of glacial acetic acid, formalin and alcohol). Long-term preservation can be done by taking photographs and by preparing models. Analysis of bitemarks in inanimate objects are not very much different from that which is used to analyze marks in the skin.
- One of the most intriguing, complex, and sometimes controversial challenges in forensic dentistry is the recognition, recovery, and analysis of bitemarks: The markings of the human dentition is objects bitten and their subsequent comparisons with the suspected biters. Most often the analysis is of bitemark injuries on the skin. Tooth markings also have been analyzed on inanimate objects associated with crime scenes, such as foods, chewing gum, styrofoam cups, cigarette butts, and the rubber seal around automobile windows; and one of the authors has testified in a case involving bitemarks on a steering wheel. The literature relating to bitemarks includes references regarding human and animal bitemarks.
- The scientific basis of bitemark analysis is rooted in the premise of the individuality of the human dentition, the belief that no two humans have identical dentitions in regard to the size, shape, and alignment of the teeth. Bitemark analysis is similar to fingerprint or DNA analyses, with one major exception. Fingerprint and DNA analyses can be expressed quantitatively as a numerical probability based on research database.

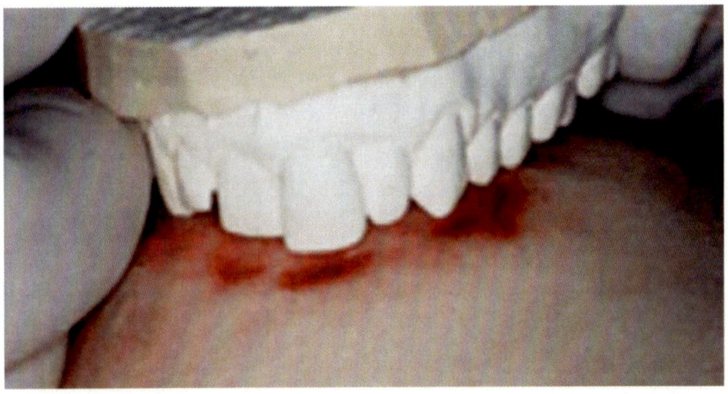

Fig. 8.23

- During the process of bitemark analysis, the unique characteristics of a suspected biter's dentition are compared with the patterns observed in the bitten skin. In a bitemark analysis, two simultaneous and opposite paths develop. The inclusive path is one in which the unique features of a suspected biter's dentition show a strong and consistent linking in a tooth-by-tooth and arch-to-arch comparison with the pattern recorded in the bitten skin. This linking is usually the strongest with a biter possessing a profoundly irregular (crooked) dentition and a bite-mark pattern in the skin that has recorded clear and distinct individual tooth pattern in the skin that has recorded clear and distinct individual tooth patterns. The exclusive path is one in which the suspected biter's dentition does not show linking with the patterns recorded in the bite-mark injury in an arch-to-arch and tooth-by-tooth analysis. In this case, the biter would be excluded as being responsible for causing the bitemark. In the authors experience, the exclusionary process is accomplished more frequently and easily than the inclusionary path.

Table 8.2: Published findings on the color changes in bruises

Time	*Camps*	*Glaister*	*Polson and Gee*	*Smith and Fiddes*
Hours: 0-24	R	V	R	R
Hours: 24-48	P/B			P/B
Day 3		B		
Days 4-5	G			G
Days 5-7		G	G	
Days 7-10	Y		G	Y
Days 8-10		Y		
Days 13-18		Resolution		
Days 14-15	Resolution		Y	Resolution
Up to day 30			Resolution	

B = blue; G = green; R = red; P/B = purple/ black; V = violet; Y = yellow (*Courtesy:* Dailey JC)

THE GUIDELINES FOR BITEMARKS

Bitemark Methodology with the Following Perspective

- There is a need for forensic dentists to agree on basic methodology used in bitemark cases so as to maximize the quality, completeness and validity of the collection and analysis of bitemark evidence. It is expected that this document is ideal to all forensic dentists. However, it represents majority opinions and has the highest level of acceptance to the largest number of odontologists. All diplomates (and other forensic odontologists) will have to make some compromises if the science of forensic odontology is to achieve the higher objective of universally agreeable methodology. There is no intention for the ABFO to mandate methods but instead to provide a list of generally accepted valid methods for this point in the development of our science. This document is not meant to stifle the development of new valid techniques that meet the criteria of the scientific method. There is every intention for the ABFO, as a credible body of experts, to present a clear and unified message as to what its members use and accept as valid methods for the collection and analysis of bitemark evidence. This document will present methods that have been agreed upon and approved as valid preservation and analysis procedures. In keeping with the commitment not to stifle the development of new methods, individuals should continue to develop new and possibly better techniques. These new techniques should be backed up by the use of accepted techniques and should satisfy the basic concepts of the scientific method.

Methods to Preserve Bitemark Evidence

Bitesite Evidence

General Considerations: It should be recognized that often the Forensic Odontologist is not involved in the initial examination and collection of the bitemark evidence. This does not necessarily preclude the ability of the Forensic Odontologist to render a valid opinion. The below listed methods are not meant to be an all encompassing list of preservation methods; however, it does list those methods that are used by the Diplomates of the ABFO. The use of other methods of documenting the Bitemark evidence should be in addition to these techniques.

Saliva Swabs of Bitesite

- Saliva swabbings of the bitesite should be obtained whenever possible. Obviously, certain circumstances

Table 8.3: Variables affecting the appearance of bruises

The structure and vascularity of the tissue injured	Bruising in the loose and highly vascular tissues around the eyes is much more pronounced than skin in areas such as the palm of the hand or the soles of the feet.
Vascular tissue over bone bruises more in children and the elderly bruise more "easily" than other generations	Because of loose delicate skin in the former and loss of subcutaneous supportive tissue in the latter.
Women bruise more easily than men	This is especially true with obese women
The victim's state of health can have an effect medications such as aspirin can increase bleeding	Hypertension, coagulation disorders, and liver dysfunction may alter the extent of bruising. Steroids can alter the dispersion rate of bruising. It has been speculated that the stress undergone by the victim may result in an endogenous release of corti costeroids, thereby delaying the healing of a bruise.
Normal color of the skin	The pigmentation may affect the observation, or missed observation of a bruise.
Mass and velocity of the impact	May have an influence of the depth and surface of injury, as well as the rate of healing.
Deep subcutaneous injury can prolong bleeding time Previous Body temperature may affect bruising at the same site Body temperature may affect the amount of bruising	May affect subsequent bruising by increasing the rate of resolution.The temperature is different on an appendage versus that over the core.
A bruise may appear at the instant of injury, or take as long as 48 hours to appear	The time of appearance is related to the time required for the extravasated blood to reach the surface. This lag time will allow antemortem bruises to appear postmortem. However, the hematoma may never become visible and only a tissue specimen would reveal its presence.
Rapidity of death after injury	May affect the presence or absence of bruising.
Bruising may occur at a site different than that of the initial injury Bruises appearing as antermortem can be created postmortem Environmental conditions may affect bruising.	Because of the movement of extravasated blood through the tissue layers.
Interpretation of color within the bruise is subjective	The observer's ability to discriminate color may be impaired (e.g. color blindness)
Ambient light may affect the appearance of the bruise.	The temperature of the light used at the time of observation.

may preclude the collection of this evidence. If the region had been washed prior to the opportunity to swab, this procedure would not be possible. If swabbing the area would damage or alter the pattern, it should either not be done or accomplished only after all other preservation methods have been employed.

- It is acceptable to use either cotton tip applicators or cigarette paper to gather this evidence. Other appropriate mediums may be used to collect this information.
- Control swabbings should be taken from other regions or portions of the object or individual that was bitten.

Photographic Documentation of the Bitesite

- The bitesite should be photographed using conventional photography and following the guidelines as described in the ABFO Bitemark Analysis Guidelines.
- The actual photographic procedures should be performed by the forensic dentist or under the odontologist's direction to insure accurate and complete documentation of the bitesite.
- Color print or slide film and back and white film should be used whenever possible.
- Color or specialty filters may be used to record the bitesite in addition to unfiltered photographs.
- Alternative methods of illumination may be used.
- Video/digital imaging may be used in addition to conventional photography.

Lighting

- Off angle lighting using a point flash is the most common form of lighting and should be utilized whenever possible.

- A light source perpendicular to the bitesite can be utilized in addition to off angle lighting; however, care should be taken to prevent light reflection from obliterating mark details in photograph due to "wash out" due to light reflection.
- A light source parallel to the bitesite can be utilized in addition to off angle lighting.
- A ring flash, natural light and/or overhead diffuse lighting can be utilized to off angle lighting.

Scale

- An ABFO No. 2 scale should be utilized whenever possible.
- The placement of the scale should follow the guidelines as established in the ABFO Bitemark Analysis Guidelines.

Impressions of Bitsite

- Victim's dental impressions
- When the bitesite is accessible to the victim's dentition impressions of the victim's teeth should be obtained.
- Would be useful if victim had bitten the assailant.
- Impressions of the Bitesite
- Impressions of the bitesite should be taken when indicated according to the ABFO Bitemark Analysis Guidelines.
- A backing material should be used to maintain the contour of the impression site.

TISSUE SPECIMEN

General Considerations

- The bitesite should be preserved when indicated following proper stabilization prior to removal.
- The resection of the tissue should follow all other evidence collecting procedures.

Tissue Fixative

- 10% Formalin is a common fixative used.
- Evidence collection of suspected dentition

Dental Records

Whenever possible the dental records of the individual should be obtained in accordance with the ABFO Bitemark Analysis Guidelines.

Photographic Documentation of the Dentition

- Photographs of the dentition should be taken by the forensic dentist or by the odontologist's direction.
- A scale such as the ABFO No. 2 scale should be utilized when using a scale in these photographs.
- Video or digital imaging can be used to document the dentition when utilized in addition to conventional photography.
- Tripods and/or focusing rails can be used at the discretion of the photographer.
- Extraoral photographs
- A frontal full face view and a view with the teeth in centric should be taken.
- Intraoral photographs
- Maxillary and mandibular occlusal views of the dentition should be taken whenever possible.
- Lateral views of the dentition may be taken.

CLINICAL EXAMINATION

Extraoral Considerations

- Maximum vertical opening and any deviations should be noted whenever possible.
- Evidence of surgery, trauma and/or facial asymmetry should be noted.
- TMJ function may be checked in addition to the previous observations.
- Muscle tone and balance may also be checked in addition to the previous observations.

Intraoral Considerations

- Missing and misaligned teeth should be noted.
- Broken and restored teeth should be noted.
- The periodontal condition and tooth mobility should be noted whenever possible.
- Previous dental charts should be reviewed if available.
- Occlusal disharmonies should be noted whenever possible.
- The tongue size and function may be noted in addition to the previous observations.
- The biteclassification may be noted in addition to the previous observations.

Dental Impressions

- Dental impressions, following the ABFO Bitemark Analysis Guidelines, should be taken by the forensic dentist or by the odontologist's direction.
- Biteexemplars should be obtained in addition to the dental impressions.

Saliva Samples

- Saliva swabbings should be obtained if appropriate. Methods of comparing bitemark evidence.

- A 1994 survey of Diplomates of the American Board of Forensic Odontology indicated that they presently use the following analytic methods in the comparison of bitemark evidence.

Generation of Overlays

- Acetate tracing directly from models of the suspect.
- Acetate tracing indirect from photocopy of model with scale.
- D-ray film overlay created from radiopaque material applied to the wax bite.
- Alternative methods
- Life-sized photos of model printed on acetate film.
- Greater than life-sized photos of models on acetate.

Test for Bitemedia

- Wax exemplars (aluwax, baseplate wax, etc.)
- Styrofoam
- Volunteer's skin
- Alternative Methods
- Fruits
- Clay

Comparison Techniques

- Acetate Tracings to life-size photos of wound
- Working study model of teeth to life-size photo of wound.
- Working study model to impression of wound or to actual victim.

Acetate overlays of teeth compared to greater than life-size photo of wound:

- Five times life-size
- Three times life-size
- Two times life-size

Technical Aids Employed for Analysis

- Transillumination of tissue
- Computer enhancement and/or digitization of mark and/or teeth
- Stereomicroscopy and/or macroscopy
- Scanning Electron Microscopy
- Videotape
- Caliper utilization for measurement

Standards for Bitemark Analytical Methods

- All Diplomates of the American Board of Forensic Odontology are responsible for being familiar with the most common analytical methods reported in this study.
- All Diplomates of the American Board of Forensic Odontology should utilize appropriate analytical methods in their analysis of the evidence.
- A list of all the evidence analyzed and the specific analytical procedures should be included in the body of the final report. All available evidence associated with the bitemark must be reviewed prior to rendering an expert opinion.
- Any new analytical methods not listed in the previously described list of analytical methods should be thoroughly explained in the body of the report. New analytical methods should be scientifically sound and duplicated by other forensic experts. New analytical methods should, if possible, be "backed up" with the use of one or more of the accepted techniques listed in thes guidelines.

BITEMARK ANALYSIS GUIDELINES

These guidelines are considered dynamic, not static, and will be modified as significant developments evolve. Careful use of these guidelines in any bitemark analysis will enhance the quality of the investigation and conclusion.

Description of Bitemark

Both in the case of a living victim or deceased individual, the odontologist should determine and record certain vital information.

Demographics

- Name of victim
- Case number
- Date of examination
- Referring agency
- Person to contact
- Age of victim
- Race of victim
- Sex of victim
- Name of examiner(s)

Location of Bitemark

- Describe anatomical location
- Describe surface contour: Flat, curved or irregular
- Describe tissue characteristics
- Underlying structure: Bone, cartilage, muscle, fat
- Skin: Relatively fixed or mobile

Shape

The shape of the bitemark should be described, e.g. essentially round, ovoid, crescent, irregular, etc.

Color

The color should be noted, e.g. red, purple, etc.

Size

Vertical and horizontal dimensions of the bitemark should be noted, preferably in the metric system.

Type of Injury

- Petechial hemorrhage
- Contusion (Ecchymosis)
- Abrasion
- Laceration
- Incision
- Avulsion
- Artifact

Other Information

- It should also be noted whether the skin surface is indented or smooth.
- At some point, the odontologist will evaluate the evidence to determine such thing as position of maxillary and mandibular arches, location and position of individual teeth, intradental characteristics, etc. This may or many not be possible at the time of initial examination and will be covered below.

Collection of Evidence from Victim

- It is assumed that evidence gathering from bitemark victims will be done with authorization from the appropriate authorities.
- It should first be determined whether the bitemark has been affected by washing, contamination, lividity, embalming, decomposition, change of position, etc.

Photography

A variety of types of photographic equipment and films may be used as described below.

- Orientation and close-up photographs should be taken.
- Photographic resolution should be of high quality.
- If color film is used, accuracy of color balance should be assured.
- Photographs of the mark should be taken with and without a scale in place.
- When the scale is used, it should be on the same plane and adjacent to the bitemark. It presently appears desirable to include a circular reference in addition to a linear scale.
- The most critical photographs should be taken in a manner that will eliminate distortion.
- In the case of a living victim, it may be beneficial to obtain serial photographs of the bitemark.

Salivary Swabbing

Whenever possible, salivary trace evidence should be collected according to recommendations of the testing laboratory.

Impressions

- Impressions should be taken of the surface of the bitemark whenever it appears that this may provide useful information.
- The impression materials used should meet. American Dental Association specifications and should be identified by name in the report.
- Suitable support should be provided for the impression material to accurately reproduce body contour.
- The material used to produce the case should accurately represent the area of impression and should be prepared according to the manufacturer's instructions.

Tissue Samples

Tissue specimens of the bitemark should be retained whenever it appears this may provide useful information.

Collection of Evidence from Suspect

Before collecting evidence from the suspect, the odontologist should ascertain that the necessary search warrant, court order or legal consent has been obtained, and should make a copy of this document part of his records. The court document or consent should be adequate to permit collection of the evidence listed below.

History

Obtain history of any dental treatment subsequent to, or in proximity to, the date of bitemark.

Photography

Whenever possible, good quality extraoral photographs should be taken, both full face and profile. Intraoral photographs preferably would include frontal view, two lateral views, occlusal view of each arch, and any additional photographs that may provide useful information. It is also useful to photograph the maximum interincisal opening with scale in place. If inanimate materials, such as foodstuffs, are used for test bites the results should be preserved photographically.

Extraoral Examination

The extraoral examination should include observation and recording of significant soft and hard tissue factors that may influence biting dynamics, such as temporomandibular joint status, facial asymmetry, muscle tone and balance. Measurement of maximal opening of the mouth should be taken, noting any deviations in opening or closing, as well as any significant occlusal disharmonies. The presence of facial scars or evidence of surgery should be noted, as well as the presence of facial hair.

Intraoral Examination

- In cases in which saliva evidence has been taken from the victim, saliva evidence should also be taken from the suspect in accordance with the specifications of the testing laboratory.
- The tongue should be examined in reference to size and function. Any abnormality such as ankyloglossia should be noted.
- The periodontal condition should be observed with particular reference to mobility and areas of inflammation or hypertrophy. Also, if anterior teeth are missing or badly broken down it should be determined how long these conditions have existed.
- It is recommended that, when feasible, a dental chart of the suspect's teeth be prepared, in order to encourage thorough study of the dentition.

Impressions

Whenever feasible, at least two impressions should be taken of each arch, using materials that meet appropriate American Dental Association specifications and are prepared according to the manufacturer's recommendations, using accepted dental impression techniques. The interocclusal relationship should be recorded.

Sample Bites

Whenever feasible, sample bites should be made into an appropriate material, simulating the type of biteunder study.

Study Casts

- Master casts should be prepared using American Dental Association approved Type II stone prepared according to manufacturer's specifications, using accepted dental techniques.
- Additional casts may be fabricated in appropriate materials for special studies. When additional models are required, they should be duplicated from master casts using accepted duplication procedures. Labeling should make it clear which master cast was utilized to produce a duplicate.
- The teeth and adjacent soft tissue areas of the master casts should not be altered by carving, trimming, marking or other alterations.

ABFO BITEMARK TERMINOLOGY GUIDELINES

These were accepted by Diplimates of the ABFO on February 13, 1995 in Seattle, Washington.

Rationale

- There is a need for forensic dentists to agree on language and terminology used in bitemark cases so as to avoid miscommunicating facts and opinions to attorneys, judges, juries and other dentists. It is not expected that this document is perfectly ideal to all forensic dentists. However, it represents majority opinions and has the highest level of acceptance to the largest number of odontologists. Please consider that major substantive changes at this time would probably make the document less representative of the group's wishes. All Diplomates (and other forensic odontologists) will have to make some compromises if the science of forensic odontology is to achieve the higher objective of universally agreeable communication.
- There is no intention for the ABFO to mandate lanugage as it is used within the body of a report or in testimony when responding to specific hypothetical questions. There is no intention to preclude the use of terms so long as they ethically and accurately communicate an odontologist's analysis and opinion.
- There is ever intention for the ABFO, as a credible body of experts, to present a clear and unified message as to what its members mean when they state a conclusion. This document will present language that has been agreed upon and approved for communicating bitemark opinions.
- Terms used to describe and interpret bitemarks
- Bitemark vs bitemark

It is the feeling of the ABFO that the meaning of the word in any of its forms is clear and there is no need for the ABFO to endorse a particular form.

Component Injuries Seen in Bitemarks

- Abrasions (scrapes), contusions (bruises), lacerations (tears), echymosis, petechiae, avulsion, indentations (depressions), erythema (redness) and punctures might be seen in bitemarks.

Characteristic (As it Pertains to Bitemarks)

Class Characteristic

A feature, trait or pattern preferentially seen in, or reflective of, a given group. For example, the finding of linear or rectangular contusions at the midline of a Bitemark arch is a class characteristic of human incisor teeth. "Incisors" represent the class in this case. The value of identifying class characteristics is that, when seen, they enable us to identify the group from which they originate. For instance, the class characteristics of incisors (rectangles) differentiates them from canines (circles or triangles). If we define the class characteristics of human bites, we can differentiate them from animal bites. Via class characteristics, we differentiate the adult from the child biteor mandibular from maxillary arch. The original term "class characteristic" was applied to toolmarks and its definition has been modified to make it more applicable to bitemarks.

Individual Characteristic

A feature, trait or pattern that represents an individual variation rather than an expected finding within a defined group. An example of this is rotated tooth. The value of individual characteristics is that they differentiate between individuals and help identify the prepetrator. The number, specificity and accurate reproduction of these individual characteristics determine the confidence level that a particular suspect made the bitemark.

Description of the Prototypical Human Bitemark

A circular or oval (doughnut) (ring-shaped) patterned injury consisting of two opposing (facing) symmetrical, U-shaped arches separated at their bases by open spaces. Following the periphery of the arches area seen of individual abrasions, contusions and/or lacerations reflecting the size, shape, arrangement and distribution of the class characteristics of the contacting surfaces of the human dentition.

Variations of the Prototypical Bitemark

Variations include additions, subtractions and distortions.

Additional Features

Central Ecchymosis (central contusion)—when found, these are caused by two possible phenomena:
- Positive pressure from the closing of teeth with disruption of small vessels.
- Negative pressure caused by suction and tongue thrusting.

Linear Abrasions, Contusions or Striations

These represent marks made by either slipping of teeth against skin or by imprinting of the lingual surfaces of teeth. The term drag marks is in common usage to describe the movement between the teeth and the skin while lingual markings is an appropriate term when the anatomy of the lingual surfaces are identified. Other acceptable descriptive terms include radial or sunburst pattern.
- Double bite—a "bitewithin a bite" occurring when skin slips after an initial contact of the teeth and then the teeth contact again a second time.
- Weave patterns of interposed clothing.
- Peripheral ecchymosis—due to excessive, confluent bruising.

Partial Bitemarks

- One-arched (half bites).
- One or few teeth.
- Unilateral (one-sided) marks—due to incomplete dentition, uneven pressure or skewed-bite.

Indistinct / Faded Bitemarks

- Fused arches—collective pressure of teeth leaves arches rings without showing individual tooth marks
- Solid-ring pattern is not apparent because erythema or contusion fills the entire center leaving a filled, discolored, circular mark.
- Closed arches—the maxillary and mandibular arch are not separate but joined at their edges.
- Latent—seen only with special imaging techniques.
- Superimposed multiple bites
- Avulsive bites.
- Unique and distinctive

Unique

This term is variably defined as either one of a kind or rare and unusual. In its most conservative interpretation the following connotations apply:
- Of such distinctiveness that no other person could have made and identical pattern.
- To the point of persuasion of individuality.
- Attributable to only one individual
- Unequalled.
- To those who use a more liberal interpretation the following would apply:
  - Unusual
  - Rare

Distinctive

- Variation from normal, unusual, infrequent.
- Not done of a kind but serves to differentiate from most others.

- Highly specific, individualized.
- Lesser degree of sepcificity than unique.

TERMS INDICATING DEGREE OF CONFIDENCE THAT AN INJURY IS A BITEMARK

Possible Bitemark

An injury showing a pattern that may or may not be caused by teeth; could be caused by other factors but biting cannot be ruled out.

Criteria

General shape and size are present but distinctive features such as tooth marks are missing, incomplete or distorted or a few marks resembling tooth marks are present but the arch configuration is missing.

Probable Bitemark

The pattern strongly suggests or supports origin from teeth but could conceivably becaused by something else.

Criteria

Pattern shows (some) (basic) (general) characteristics of teeth arranged around arches.

Definite Bitemark

There is no reasonable doubt that teeth created the pattern; other possibilities were considered and excluded.

Criteria

Pattern conclusively illustrates (classic features) (all the characteristics) (typical class characteristics) of dental arches and human teeth in proper arrangement so that it is recognizable as an impression of the human dentition.

Table 8.4: Terms used to indicate that an injury is a bitemark

Ordinate Ranking of terms	*Connotation*
Definite positively	No doubt in my mind it is a bitemark
Reasonable medical certainty	Virtual certainty; allows for the possibility of another cause, however remote
Highly probable probable possible similar to consistent with	More likely than not
Conceiveable may or may not be cannot be ruled out cannot be excluded unlikely	Such a mark could have been produced by teeth but not necessarily and could have been created by something else; no commitment to likelihood
Inconsistent improbable incompatible excluded	Less likely than not no doubt in my mind it is not a bitemark; represents something else
Impossible indeterminable shouldn't be used insufficient	Pattern shows insufficient characterization to comment on teeth as a cause

Point

- A singular unit or feature available for comparison or evaluation
- An area attributable to a tooth
- A way of counting features

Concordant Point

- Point seen in both the bitemark and the suspect(s') exemplars
- Corresponding feature
- Comparable element
- Unit of similarity
- Matching point

Area of Comparison

- A dynamic or specific region to be compared.
- A complex or pattern made up of a conglomerate of several points or a group of features.

Match

- Nonspecific term indicating some degree of concordance between a single feature, combination of features or a whole case.
- An expression of similarity without stating degree of probability or specificity.

Consistent (Compatible)

Synonymous to "match", a similarity is present but specificity is unstated.

Possible Biter

- Could have done it; may or may not have.
- Teeth like the suspect's could be expected to create a mark like the one examined but so could other dentitions.

Probable Biter

Suspect most likely made the bite; most people in the population could not leave such a mark.

Criteria

Bitemark shows some degree of specificity to the individual suspect's teeth by virtue of a sufficient number of concordant points including some corresponding individual characteristics. There is an absence of any unexplainable discrepancies.

Reasonable Medical Certainty

- Highest order of certainty that suspect made the bite.
- The investigator is confident that the suspect made the mark.
- Perpetrator is identified for all practical and reasonable purposes by the bitemark.
- Any expert with similar training and experience, evaluating the same evidence should come to the same conclusion of certainty.
- Any other opinion would be unreasonable.

Criteria

There is a concordance of sufficient distinctive, individual characteristics to confer (virtual) uniqueness within the population under consideration. There is absence of any unexplainable discrepancies.

ABFO Standards for Bitemark Terminology

- The following list of Bitemark Terminology Standards have been accepted by the American Board of Forensic Odontology.
- Terms assuring unconditional identification of a perpetrator, without doubt, on the basis of an epidermal bitemark and an open population is not sanctioned as a final conclusion.
- Terms used in a different manner from the recommended guidelines should be explained in the body of a report or in testimony.
- Certain terms have been used in a nonuniform manner by odontologists. To prevent miscommunication, the following terms, if used as a conclusion in a report or in testimony, should be explained
  - Match; positive match
  - Consistent with
  - Compatible with
  - Unique

The following terms should not be used to describe bitemarks

- Suck mark (20% of diplomates still use this antiquated term).
- Incised wound

All boarded forensic odontologists are responsible for being familiar with the standards set forth in this document.

GUIDELINES FOR REPORT WRITING

General Comments

- The following outline lists recommended components of a forensic report regarding a bitemark analysis. This is a continuation of previous guidelines established by the ABFO and follows a natural progression of events as we have existing terminology guidelines and standards already established. It is the hope that these report-writing guidelines will establish a uniform way of using the terminology guidelines/ standards to present expert opinions in a logical, complete and defendable manner.
- This report protocol is fairly standard for forensic reports and would include when and who was the initial contact and what we were requested to do.
- The next section is an inventory of the evidence that is available for analysis. There are two selections and the odontologist would use the one that is appropriate. The only difference between the two is that if the odontologist collects the evidence then a description of the evidence collection procedures should be included in the report. If the odontologist does not collect the material then a simple inventory would suffice. It is the responsibility of the person that collected the information to demonstrate that the evidence was collected properly and met the current ABFO guidelines and standards. If items listed here are not available or were not obtained, the reason for theri omission should be noted.
- The ABFO Bitemark Terminology Guidelines and Standards should be followed in all written communications regarding the evidence, analysis and opinions. This will eliminate a lot of confusion and misunderstanding concerning the expert's opinions.
- The order in which the information is presented is important in laying a sound foundation for the stated opinion. The analysis of the injury should include the expert's opinion concerning the degree of certainty that it is a bitemark. Following this is a description of the dentition that will be used for the comparison. Details of the comparison procedures should follow the description of the dentition. Finally, the expert's opinion as to the degree of certainty that there is a link (or non-link) between the dentition and the bitemark should be stated clearly and follow the recommended terminology as noted in the ABFO Bitemark Terminology Guidelines.

- These guidelines are not static and will be changed as new techniques and advances are made in the field of Forensic Odontology.
- The Diplomates of the American Board of Forensic Odontology, Inc. approved these Guidelines, on February 15, 1999.
- Suggested Components of a Forensic Odonotology Report: Bitemarks.

Introduction

- When and Who contacted you requesting services.
- Inventory of Evidence Received (if not involved directly with the evidence collection).

Injury Evidence

- # and type of photographs
- # and type of impressions
- # and type of casts
- Description of tissue samples and how they were preserved and packaged

Dentition Evidence

- Description of inter- and extraoral examination
- # and type of photographs
- # and type of wax bites/impressions
- # and type of impressions
- # and type of casts

OR

Evidence collection procedures (if involved directly with the evidence collection)

- Description of evidence collection procedures in chronological order (both for injury and dentition)
- Itemized list of the types and quantity of evidence collected

Analysis of Injury Evidence

- Description of the injury using ABFO Bitemark Terminology Guidelines
- Appropriate embedded annotated images
- Description of the quality of the evidence. (photographic distortion? etc.) (If Appropriate)
- Description of analytical procedures used to analyze the injury (trans, microscopy, etc.)
- Opinions as to the degree of certainty that the injury is a bitemark (using guidelines and standards) and justification for this degree of certainty.

Analysis of Dentition

- Description of the dentition(s) being compared to the injury
- Appropriate embedded annotated images
- Description of the evidence taken of the dentition (if appropriate)
- Description of procedures used to prepare evidence for comparison to the bitemark
- Define dental numbering system used in the report.

Comparison Procedures

Description of the procedures utilized to compare the dentition to the bitemark using the ABFO Bitemark Methodology Guidelines and Standards.

Opinions

- Description of the degree of certainty for link between the dentition and the bitemark using the ABFO Bitemark Terminology Guidelines and Standards with justification for this degree of certainty.
- Appropriate embedded annotated images.

HIV AND BITES

- The transmission of the human immunodeficiency virus via human biteis important to number of distinct groups. The first group are those who are likely to be bitten as an occupational risk, such as police officers, correctional officers, medical personnel and other working in an institutional setting. Another group are represented by the victims and perpetrators of crimes involving biting—both in attack and defense situations. The possibility of these bites transmitting a potentially fatal disease is of interest to the physicians who treat such patients and the legal system who may have to deal with the repercussions of such a transmission. A biteinjury which transmitted HIV to the recipient could be classed as assault with a deadly weapon.
- Other diseases have been transmitted by bitting such as syphilis and hepatitis B. Case examples do exist which demonstrate the potential for HIV to be transmitted via a bite.
- Bites have been described to occur in a number of situations, including overtly aggressive behavious (violent and sexual attacks), accidental bites (e.g. those associated with sports and medical treatment) and sexual activity. The site of a biteis an important variable in the risk of infection. Male victims of bites are most frequently bitten on the hand, arm and shoulder; female victims are most frequently bitten on the breast, genitalia, leg or arm. The distribution of bites are: For hand and upper extremities 60-75%, for head of neck 15-20%, for trunk 10-20%, for lower extremities 5% and for other sites 5-10% there is a bias introduced by the fact that figures.

- Relate only to those individuals who sought treatment. Failure to attend could be motivated by the severity of the injury, inadequate self-treatment or if the individual was attacked as part of a violent crime. Many individuals do not seek treatment for human bites due to embarrassement and legal repercussions.
- The reported infection rate of human bites varies. The infection rate for a biteof the hand was 28% compared to only 4% for bites to the facial area. Human bites have a higher incidence of infection than any other bitetype such as dog or cat.
- The hand, of all potential bitesites, is the most likely to have and infective sequel, especially if the injury involves the metcarpophalangeal joint. This kind of injury is most likely to occur in a "clenched first" situation. This typically occurs when the attacker strikes and hits the victim in the mouth and causes a laceration from the teeth. In the clenched fist injury, a laceration of roughly 5 mm occurs, typically in the third MCP joint (normally the most prominent), which looks superficial and benign. Typically, the patient will extend their hand to examine the injury and in the process create a deep inoculum of oral bacteria that enter the wound.

Nature of Bites

Bites can be described in an ascending scale of severity, beginning with petechial hemorrhage (errythema), contusion (ecchymosis), abrasion, laceration (incision), and ending with avulsion. The severity of the biteinjury is one factor that is likely to increase the chance of HIV transmission. HIV is a predominately blood transmitted virus. So, in order to access the victims blood, a bitemust at least break the skin—hence an abrasion or more sever injury. Consideration must also be given to skin that is already broken. For example, skin with a previous injury or pathological lesion that suffers a superficial bite may allow saliva or oral blood to contact the biterecipients' blood.

Prevalence of HIV

- The presence of HIV in saliva has been examined by many investigators. Suggested a decline in the relative HIV presence in saliva as the disease progresses. The decreasing viral load, with increasing disease progression, is explained by the reduction in the number of immune products available, and hence the number of antibodies available for test diagnosis. 70% of patients and 93% of patients with AIDS-related compexes had salivary antibodies to HTLV-III , HIV isolated from 21% of the saliva samples versus of the blood samples, in the presenc eof periodontal disease, a source of oral blood.
- The oral cavity may contain blood, and saliva can become contaminated with this blood. Presence of blood would indirectly indicate the presence of such microlesions. After activities such as teeth brushing, eating or passionate kissing the blood quantity in saliva increases significantly. It is also true that many dental procedures such as supra and subgingival scaling, cavity preparations and impressions are likely to produce the same increase in salivary blood load.
- Researchers discovered the presence of retrovirus like particles from major salivary glands, another possible indication of the likelihood of saliva containing HIV. The low viral detection from saliva in terms of the presence of HIV inhibiting factors. "Saliva inhibits HIV-1 infectivity" protein in saliva had significant anti- retroviral activity and that this may be important in the low transmission rate of HIV via the oral route. Specific IgA antibody exists in saliva to HIV may be more transmissible via the salivary route. There are several mechanisms at work inhibiting HIV in saliva.
- Despite ample evidence for anti-HIV factors in saliva, the extent to which they operate *in vivo* is unknown, viral quantity in saliva is low or is supplemented by the presence of blood contamination. The source of this blood may be from undetectable microlesions, trauma or periodontal disease. The saliva may not appear blood stained on visual inspection but can still contain blood. Several oral diseases are aassociated with AIDS and HIV. These include acute ulcerative gingivitis and periodontitis (ANUG, ANUP), Kaposis' sarcoma and hairy leukoplakia. These oral conditions are likely to cause intraoral bleeding, and hence the risk of infection from those individuals demonstrating these conditions is likely to be increased. Considering the oral cavity as potentially containing HIV—whether from blood or saliva sources allows a simpler analysis of the transmission risk.

CHAPTER 9

Ethics

CODE OF ETHICS

- From constitution bye laws and code of ethics of "The Indian Dental Association" as amended upto January 31, 1988.
- In order that the dignity and honor of the dental profession may be upheld, its standards exalted, its sphere of usefulness extended and the advancement of dental science promoted and that the members of the Indian Dental Association may understand more clearly their duties and obligations to the dental profession, to their patients, and to the community at large, the following Code of Ethics is prescribed.

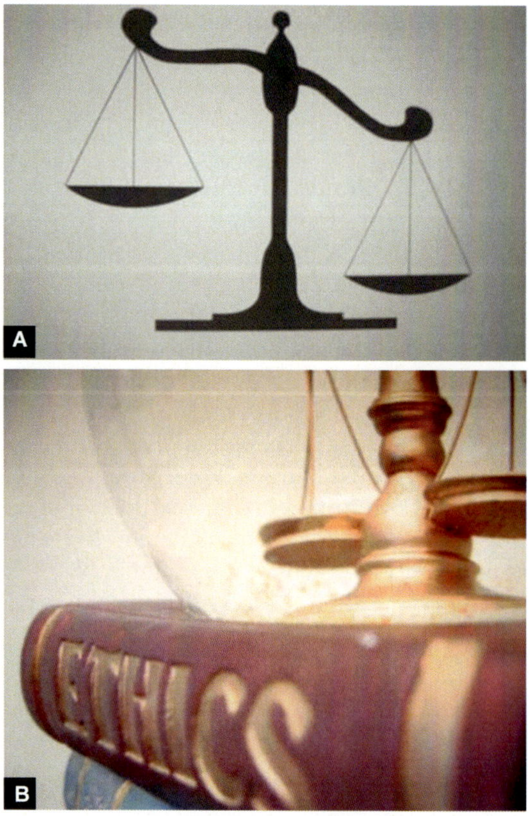

Figs 9.1A and B

Section 1

It is the duty of every dentist, and it shall be incumbent upon every member of this Association to govern his department in accordance with the underlying principles which have motivated the formulation of the code. It is not assumed that the following chapter cover the whole field of dental ethics, the dentist is charged with many duties and obligations in addition to those set forth herein. Briefly the "Golden Rule" should be conscientiously applied by every member of the dental profession.

Section 2

It is unprofessional for a dentist to advertise by handbills, posters, circulars, cards and signs, or in newspapers or in publications, calling attention to special methods of practice or claiming excellence over other practitioners, or touse display advertisements of any kind. It is also unprofessional to publish reports of cases or certificates in the public prints. This does not exclude a practitioner, either from using professional cards of the suitable size with name, titles, address and telephone number printed in modest type of having the same character of card in a newspaper at the time of commencement of practice or change of address for not more than three insertions at a time. Neither does it prevent a practitioner who confines himself to a specialty—from merely announcing his specialty on his professional card.

Section 3

It is unprofessional for dentists to pay or accept commission on fees for professional services, or for radiograms, or on prescriptions of other articles supplied to patients by pharmacists or others.

Section 4

One dentist should not disparage the services of another to a patient. Criticism of operations which are apparently defective may be unjust through lack of knowledge of the conditions under which they were performed. But the welfare of the patient is paramount to every other consideration, and should be conserved to the utmost of the practitioner's ability. If he finds indisputable evidence that a patient is suffering from previous faulty treatment, it is his duty to institute correct treatment at once, doing it with as little comment as possible and in such manner as to avoid reflection on his predecessor.

Section 5

If a dentist is consulted in an emergency by the patient of another practitioner who is temporarily absent from his office, or by a patient who is away from home, the duty of the dentist so consulted is to relieve the patient of any immediate disability by temporary service only, and then refer the patient back to the regular dentist.

Section 6

When a dentist is called in consultation by fellow practitioner, he should hold the discussions in the consultation as confidential, and under no circumstances should he accept charge of the case without the request of the dentist who has been attending it.

Section 7

It is unethical for dentists to connive at or aid in illegal practice by others. It is their duty to expose such persons without fear or favor. Dentists shall call to the attention of the committee of Ethics of Indian Dental Association, illegal, corrupt or dishonest conduct on the part of any member of the dental profession.

Section 8

It is unethical for dentists to give testimonials directly or indirectly, concerning the supposed virtue of secret therapeutic agent or medicines or to promise radical cures by employing secret methods of treatment.

Section 9

The dentist should be morally, mentally and physically clean. He should be honest in all his dealings with his fellow men, as comforts with the honor and dignity of a cultured and professional gentlemen.

JURISPRUDENCE ISSUES IN FORENSIC ODONTOLOGY

- The practice of forensic odontology requires an understanting of the judicial system.
- The frame work supporting the acceptance or refusal of dental expert testimony in the legal arena
- Common questions dentists ask about their role as an expert
- How certain scientific issues (e.g. bitemark analysis) should be described in court.
- How the legal profession views malpractice regarding expert witnesses.

CHAPTER 10

Age Estimation by Teeth

The ageing of unknown human remains is based upon a detailed knowledge of biological changes that occur during development, growth and maturation. This chapter is confined to approaches within the expertise of the forensic odontologist. It is convenient to look at the problem from four standpoints:

- Changes occurring during fetal life
- Those associated with the period around birth
- Those from birth to the onset of the third decade
- Those from young adulthood to old age

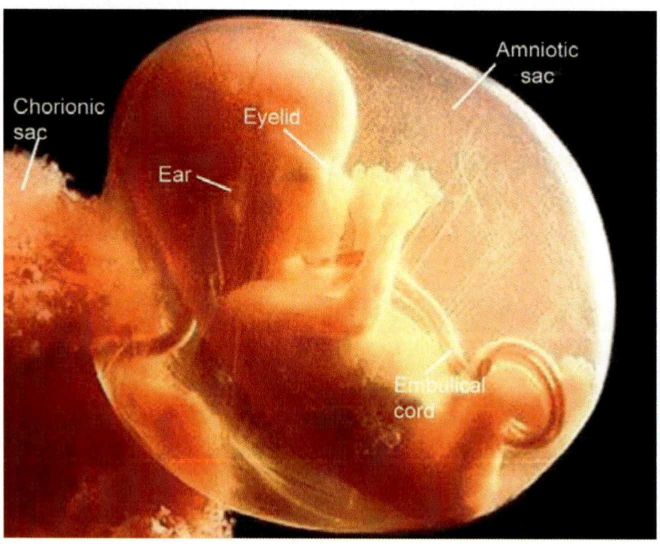

Fig. 10.1

PRENATAL DEVELOPMENT

- The forensic dentist is rarely involved in the ageing of the unborn fetus, but occasionally premature births or abortion specimens may have to be aged.
- *The human fetus:* The fist signs of tooth development in man are seen at about six weeks of intra-uterine life when the downgrowths of the oral epithelium (the dental laminae) develop. Individual tooth germs differentiate at the future sites of the deciduous teeth, and later the permanent molars, but it is not until about 16 weeks that the first of these, the deciduous incisors, begin to mineralize.

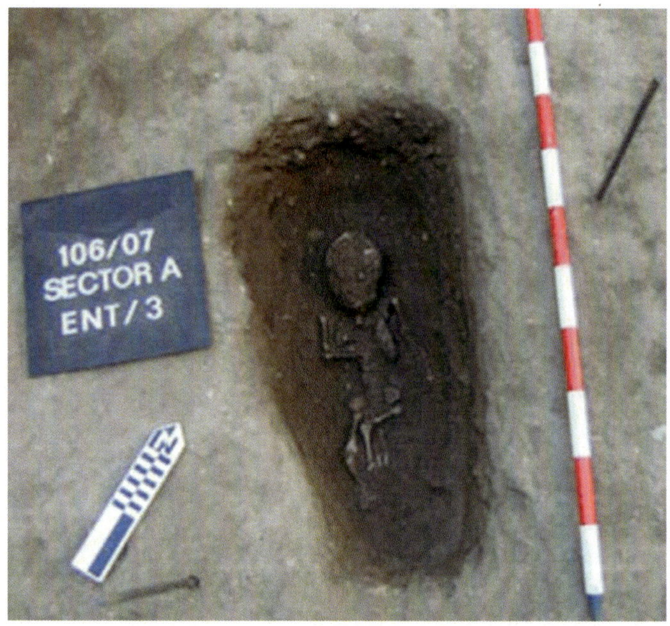

Fig. 10.2

- *Jaw of twenty-six week fetus:* Mandible of an unborn human fetus begun to mineralize. The process is well-advanced in the anterior teeth, and in the crypt for the first deciduous molar the mineralized outline of two cusps can be seen. In the crypt for the second deciduous molar initial mineralization of one cusp is just visible, and as this process starts at about six months of intrauterine life this child was about 26 weeks from conception to the time of death. Posterior to the crypt for the second deciduous molar is the early formation of the crypt for the first permanent molar. No evidence of mineralization is seen in this tooth at this stage. Fetal skeletons may also be aged from the lengths of certain of the long bones and the mandible, and tables of expected dimensions are available.

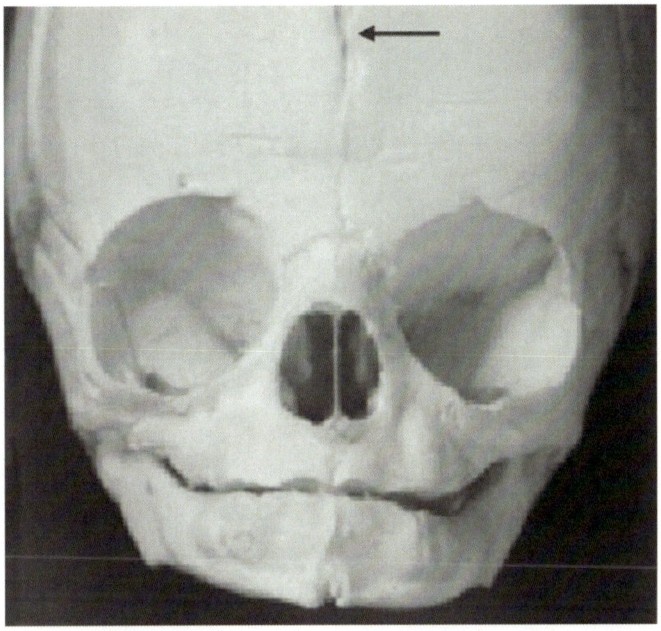

Fig. 10.3

- *Jaw of thirty week fetus:* Mineralization of the anterior teeth is now more obvious and the crown in the incisor region on the right of the picture is about three-fifths complete. The crypt of the lower second deciduous molar contains a tooth with five cusps which are beginning to mineralize, but they are widely separated. In the first deciduous molar, the cusps have begun to fuse together but are still not completely united. There is no evidence of mineralization in the first permanent molar. These features indicate that this fetus has not yet reached full-term and is probably about 30 weeks from conception.

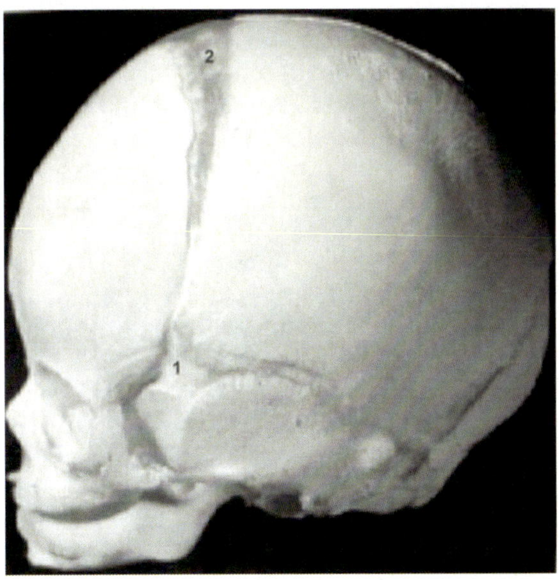

Fig. 10.4

- *Histology:* Standard radiographs of fetal material may sometimes be difficult to interpret because the extent of mineralization may not be clearly seen. Ageing may be confirmed from sections through the jaw and tooth so that the stage of hard tissue formation may be studied. In this section through a molar tooth the papilla can be seen and above it the mineralizing dentine. The enamel matrix is not yet mature and has not been lost during the demineralization procedure. Active ameloblasts are present at the periphery of the enamel matrix indicating that the outline of the crown is not yet complete. As this section is of the mesiolingual cusp of a deciduous lower molar, the age at death is probably about eight months from conception. Because the organic component in the enamel decreases during maturation, another method of ageing the fetus and newborn is to estimate biochemically the amount of organic material present and to relate this information to developing teeth of known maturity.

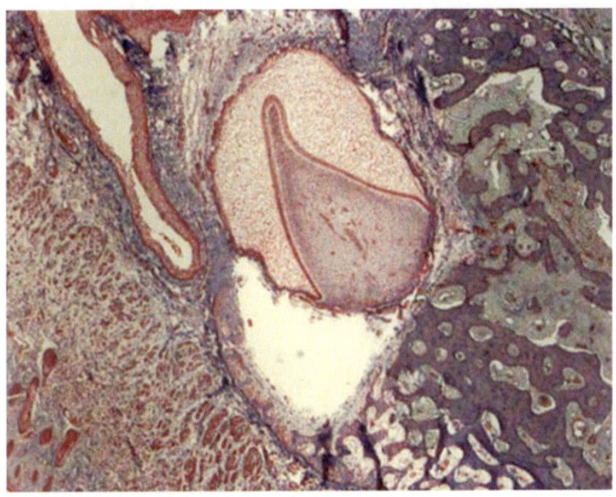

Fig. 10.5

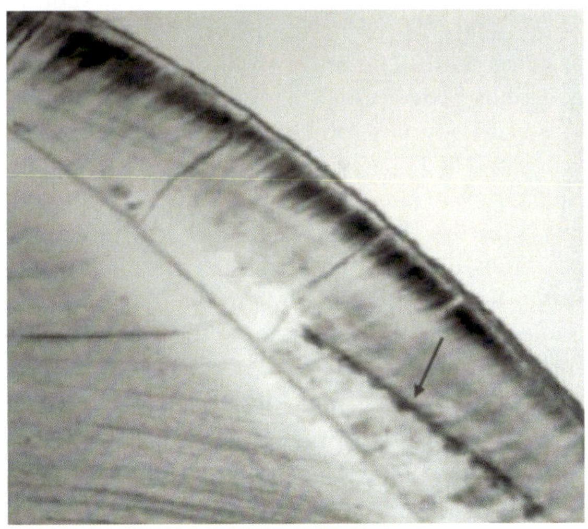

Fig. 10.6

AGE DETERMINATION IN THE NEWBORN

- During birth the fetal skull has to be compressed so that it can pass down the birth canal. This is possible because the bones of the vault are spaced out with connective tissue which forms the fontanelles. These are replaced by bone in the period after birth so that the sutures are formed.

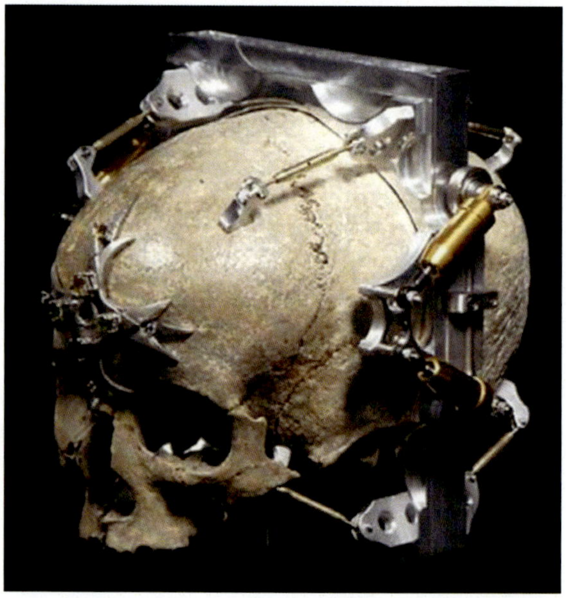

Fig. 10.7

- *Jaws of the newborn child:* The absence of erupted teeth in the normal child suggests that the age is less than six months, but eruption times are notoriously variable. It is not unknown for teeth (usually lower incisors) to be erupted at birth, and these are referred to as neonatal teeth. The orbits are relatively well-developed at this stage, whilst the jaws are of minimum bone height as they are not yet required to support erupted teeth. The brain and hence the cranial vault are proportionally large so that the face of the newborn appears to be diminutive when compared with the total size of the baby's head.
- *Radiograph of mandible:* This radiograph of the lower jaw at birth shows several features which are useful in age estimation. The cusps of the first deciduous molar have mineralized and have fused producing a continuous occlusal surface. In the second deciduous molar some of the cusps have fused but there is still no continuity across the whole of the occlusal surface. Within the crypt of the first permanent molar one of the mesial cusps has started to mineralize indicating a newborn infant.

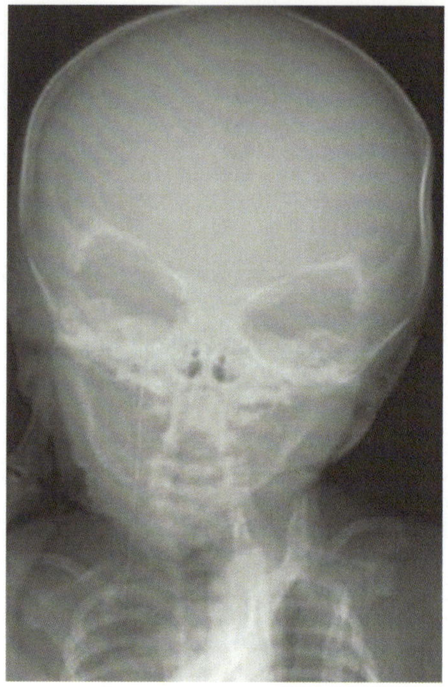

Fig. 10.8

Stillborn Infants

- It is frequently important for medicolegal reasons to determine whether the body of an infant is that of a newborn or a stillborn child. If the soft tissues are reasonably intact it may be possible, from the changes occurring at birth in the lungs, heart and surrounding vessels, to determine whether the child actually had an independent existence. If the soft tissues have been destroyed and only skeletal material is available, this may be much more difficult.
- *Neonatal line:* Some of the teeth begin their development before birth and growth continues through birth into the neonatal period. When the child is born the physiological upset results in a change in metabolic activity of the cells producing the hard tissues of the tooth. An accentuated growth or incremental line frequently results, in both the enamel and the dentine. In this microscopic ground section of the deciduous tooth of a child, such an accentuated incremental line can be seen in the outer enamel dividing the prenatal enamel nearest to the dentine from the postnatal enamel nearest to the surface of the tooth. For such a neonatal line to be clearly visible with the light microscope, a reasonable thickness of postnatal enamel has to be produced. In practice, this means that the method can be used only if the child survives for about three weeks after birth.

AGE DETERMINATION DURING THE FIRST TWO DECADES OF LIFE

- During the first six months of the life no teeth are clinically visible in the baby's mouth. This radiograph of the mandible suggests that the deciduous incisor crowns are now complete and the crown of the first molar is well on its way to completion. The occlusal surface of the second deciduous molar is continuous, and there is a mineralized cusp tip visible in the mesial part of the first permanent molar. This degree of development of the dentition would indicate an age of around three months after birth.
- *Histological studies:* This section was taken from where considerable putrefaction has taken place and staining is difficult, the cell outlines in the pulp, periodontal ligament and bone marrow spaces can still be seen.

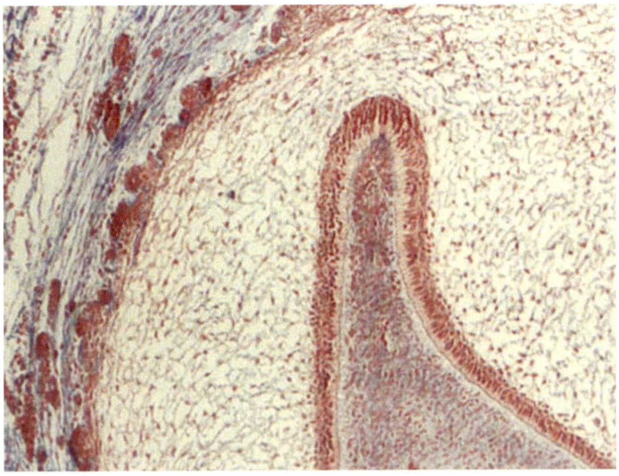

Fig. 10.9

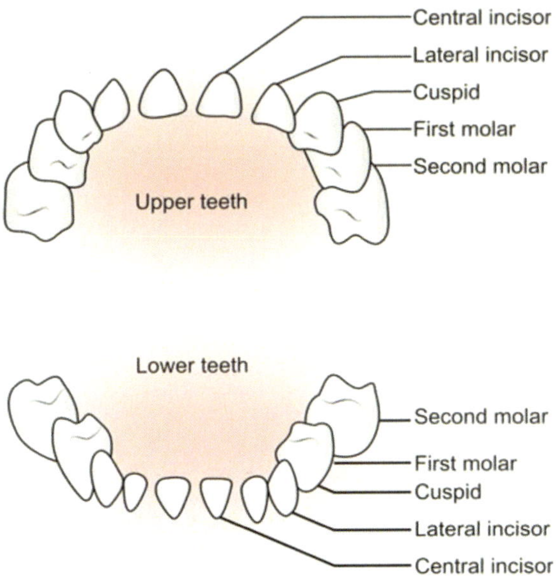

Fig. 10.10

Ageing of an unknown body from the dentition is done first by using the eruption status of the teeth, and second by studying the degree of their development. This tooth is the lower central incisor and the degree of root development confirms the age of three months after birth. Age estimation would be possible using radiographs of the long bones and epiphyses, but may also be confirmed by an examination of the dentition.

- *Permanent teeth:* The first permanent teeth to erupt into the oral cavity and come into full occlusion are the first molars. They are followed about six months to a year later by the eruption of first the lower and then the upper central incisors. In this skull the permanent upper central incisors have not yet reached the occlusal plane. The deciduous lateral incisors, canines and molars are still present and the age would be around seven years. A radiograph of the molar region showed the presence of a developing second permanent molar, the crown of which was virtually complete, confirming the age of seven to eight years.

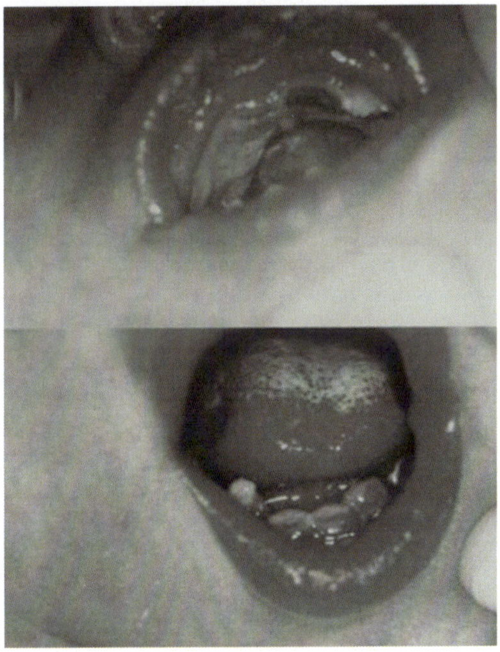

Fig. 10.11

- *Root resorption in the mixed dentition:* The stage where both deciduous and permanent teeth are present together is known as the mixed dentition stage. As time progresses the deciduous teeth will resorb and be exfoliated, thus allowing the permanent teeth below them to erupt into occlusion. The degree of resorption of the root of the deciduous tooth may therefore be a useful age indicator. Variations in resorption of the deciduous teeth occur depending upon the presence or absence of their permanent successors. It is important that the whole dentition be examined in detail so that ageing is based on as many features as possible.

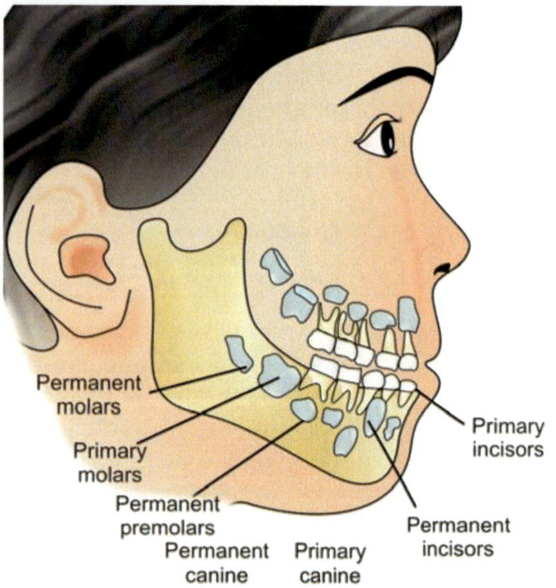

Fig. 10.12

- *Teenage dentition:* In this skeleton the second molars have erupted into occlusion and the premolars are erupting and reaching their functional position. The degree of accuracy of ageing becomes less in older individuals, and from an examination of clinically visible teeth it would only be possible to age this skull at somewhere between 10 and 13 years. As in previous examples, it is advisable to take radiographs so that the position and degree of development of all the teeth including their roots can be ascertained.
- *The wisdom teeth:* Although the timing of eruption of the wisdom teeth may be variable, the process of development of the roots is a more reliable guide to age.

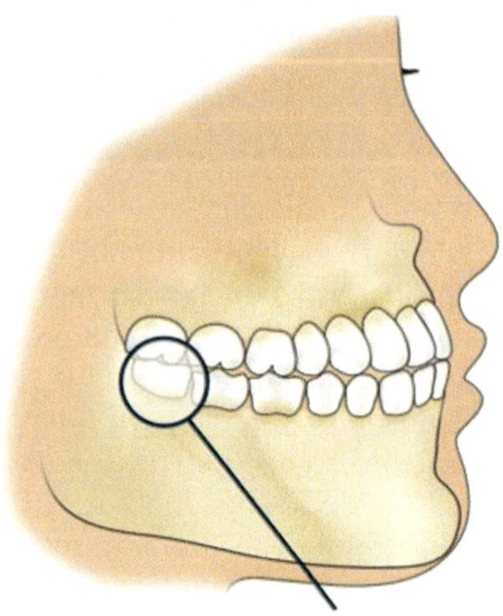

Fig. 10.13

When a tooth erupts, the root is about two-thirds complete, and it has been shown that the root apices are always complete at around age 23 to 24 years. In this example the roots are approximately half formed, indicating that the individual was around 17 years of age. The completion of the apices of the third molar mark the point after which age estimation from development and eruption of the teeth is no longer a useful method.

- *Tooth sockets:* An unknown body may be aged from the stages of development and eruption of the teeth, but there may also be evidence of the stage of tooth development in the skeleton even when the teeth are not present. In this case the mandible of a young adult was found separated from the remainder of the body and the lower third molar had been lost. Examination of the base of the socket of the two roots shows that there are flattened areas of bone suggesting that the third molar tooth had not completed its development. This fragment was aged from this feature alone as belonging to a person of approximately 22 years.

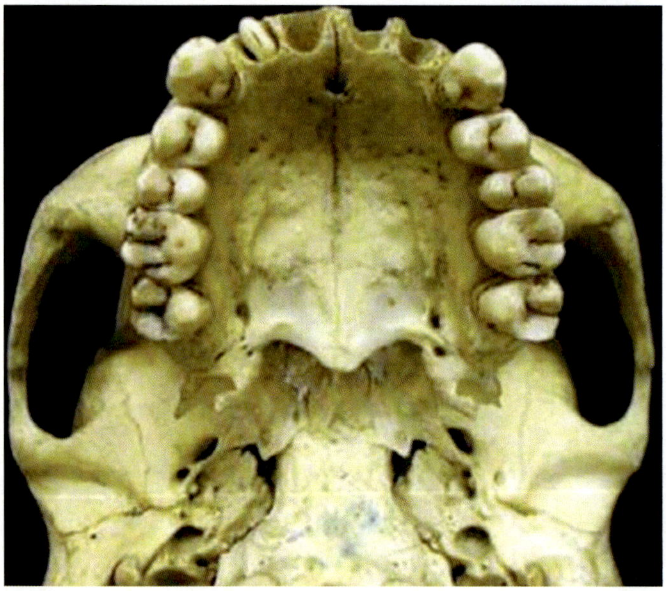

Fig. 10.14

AGE DETERMINATION AFTER THE FIRST TWO DECADES OF LIFE

- Once the development of crowns and roots is completed and the teeth are in functional occlusion, age determination using dental findings becomes more difficult. However, ageing by long bone criteria or closure of sutures and synchondroses is also subject to variation so dental estimates of age are still extremely useful in forensic investigations. After the age of about

24 years dental estimates depend upon subtle changes in the teeth which are dependent not only upon increasing age but also upon the effects of wear and tear.

- *Translucent apices:* Skeletons older than 24 years at death become increasingly difficult to age and usually require preparation of sections through the teeth. If such specialized techniques are not available, useful information may be obtained by cutting through the mandible or maxilla alongside a standing permanent tooth. In this case the mandible has been sectioned immediately next to the distal surface of a lower canine. The root of the tooth is not uniformly opaque throughout its length, there being a degree of translucency near to the apex. This change is related to age rather than to pathology in the tooth. The apical translucency is minimal or absent in a 20-year-old but involves at least half of the root of the tooth in someone aged 70 years.
- *Age determination using tooth sections:* Gustapson described a method for ageing the dead which was based upon changes occurring in the teeth as age progresses. He awarded arbitrary points to the degree of occlusal wear (i), the amount of secondary dentine in the pulp chamber (ii), the level of the gum attachment around the neck of the tooth (iii), the extent of translucent or sclerotic apical dentine (iv), the amount of secondary cementum at the apex (v) and the extent of resorption of the apex. This latter feature has been shown to be very unreliable and is no longer used.

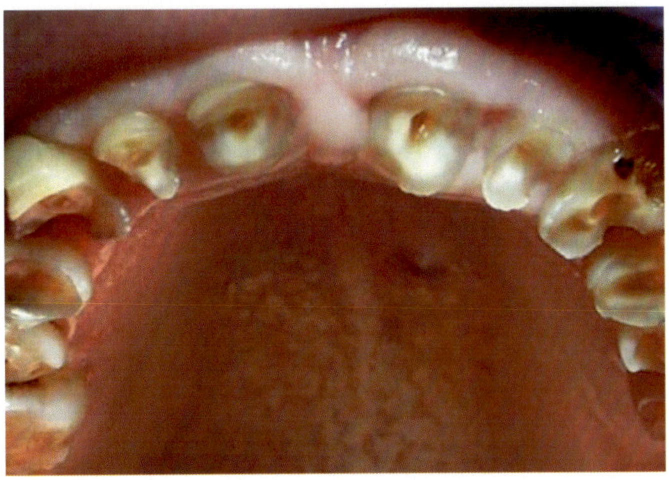

Fig. 10.15

- If any of these features is unchanged from the situation in a tooth which has recently completed its development then no points are awarded. Minimal change, for example enamel wear but not extending to dentine is awarded one point. Severe change, for example translucency extending halfway up the root, is awarded three points. The points awarded to each feature are added and the total compared with a regression line prepared from teeth of known age. The method requires considerable expertise and should be attempted only by a dentist practiced in its use.

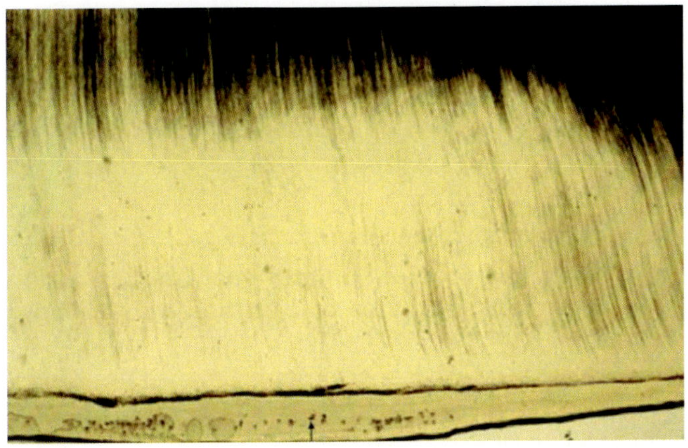

Fig. 10.16

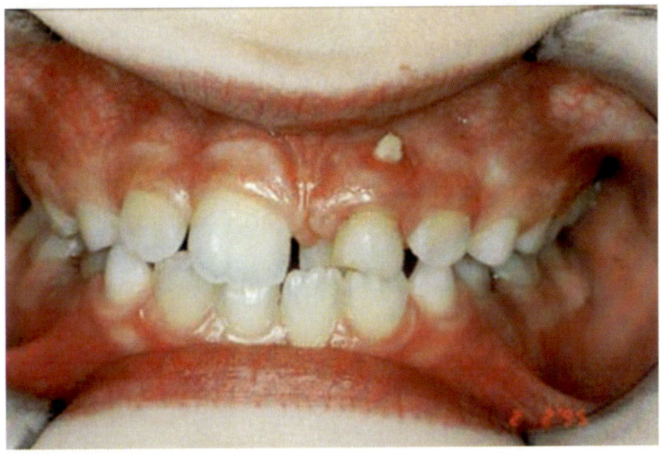

Fig. 10.17

- *Translucent apical dentine:* The most reliable change in ageing teeth appears to be the extent of sclerotic or translucent apical dentine. Various methods have been suggested to quantify this phenomenon, one of them uses sections through the teeth 1 mm in thickness and another uses accurate measurement of the translucent area rather than awarding points based on its extent. This latter method used alone on one tooth is said to be capable of estimating age to within five years in about 60 percent of cases. However, further studies of this technique are necessary because it has recently been shown that the translucent zone is not symmetrical in the root apex, so the determined age may depend upon the direction in which the tooth is sectioned.

CHAPTER 11

Scientific Methods of Identification

INTRODUCTION

It involves the cooperation and coordination of law enforcement officials, forensic pathologists, forensic odontologists, forensic anthropologists, serologists, criminalists, and other specialists as deemed necessary.

IDENTIFICATION PARAMETERS

Legal certification of an individual's identity is based on a number of parameters most of which are centered about the individual's appearance and personal effects. As such, many persons are buried or cremated based on a visual identification or other presumptive identification methods. A positive identification is preferred to a presumptive identification. Positive identifications traditionally involve a comparison of pre- and postmortem data which are considered unique to the individual. These methods include: (i) Dental comparisons, (ii) Fingerprints, palm prints, and footprints (iii) DNA identification, and (iv) Radiographic superimpositions (vertebrae, cranial structures including frontal sinuses, pelvic structures, bone trabeculae, and prostheses). Presumptive identifications which include visual recognition, personal effects, serology, anthropometric data, and medical but rather present a series of general or class characteristics which may exclude others based on race, sex, build, age, blood group, etc. Most positive identifications today are based on dental examinations and fingerprints and are fundamental procedures in medicolegal death investigations including mass disasters. The development of DNA analysis is providing investigators with yet another very important tool in the identification process.

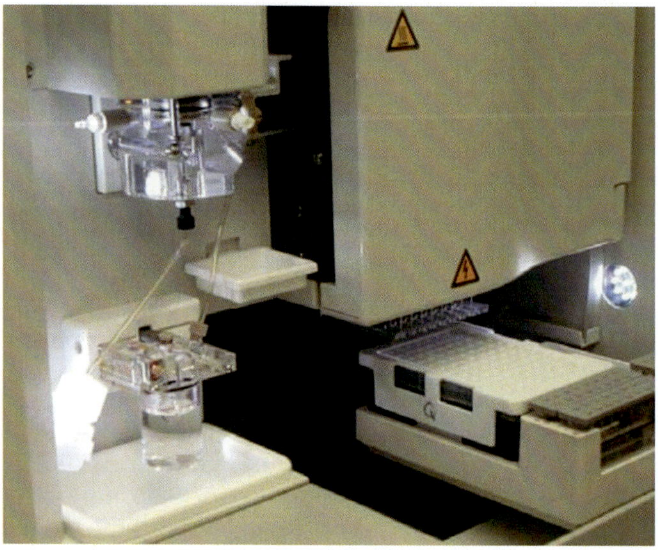

Fig. 11.1

FORENSIC ODONTOLOGY

- Forensic odontology has three major areas of utilization: (i) Diagnostic and therapeutic examination and evaluation of injuries of jaws, teeth, and oral soft tissues, (ii) The identification of individuals, especially casualties in criminal investigations and/or mass disasters, and (iii) Identification, examination, and

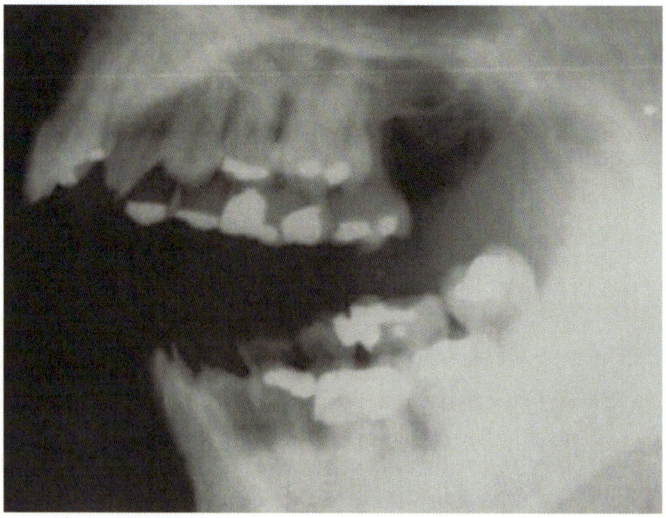

Fig. 11.2

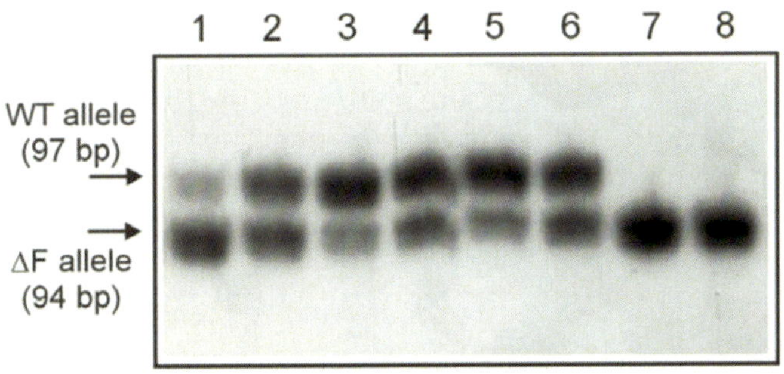

Fig. 11.3

evaluation of bitemarks which occur with some frequency in sexual assaults, child abuse cases, and in personal defense situations.

- The odontological identification examination of a decedent is based on a systematic comparison of the pre- and postmortem dental characteristics of the individual based on the dental record and supporting radiographs (apical films, panographs and medical skull films). A variety of techniques can be used to narrow the search and are based on presumptive identification data which are often sorted with computer assistance. The final identification is based on validation of the premortem data and their comparison with the postmortem data. This comparison can be complicated by any attending trauma or by the absence of adequate premortem dental information. This increasing circumstance complicates dental identification efforts especially when computerized databases are used such as CAPMI (computerized assisted postmortem identification system) which tabulates restorations and missing teeth as sorting parameters.
- A variety of techniques are used to assist in the identification issue. These include (i) Amino acid racemization studies, especially aspartic acid, (ii) Incremental line and other histology studies, (iii) Scanning electron microscopy with and without energy—dispersive X-ray analysis, (iv) Metal ratio analysis in bone and teeth, (v) Serology studies for blood groups, serum proteins, and polymorphic enzymes, and (vi) Most recently, DNA analyses.

ANCILLARY TECHNOLOGIES

Age Determinants

- Aspartic acid racemization has been used for age estimation based on its presence in human. This technology applied to dental forensic issues is a spinoff of paleontology studies on fossil bone and shells. Most protein components in the body consist of L-amino acids, whereas D-amino acids are believed to have a slower metabolic turnover and subsequently a slower decomposition rate. Aspartic acid has the highest racemization rate of all of the amino acids. In 1976, Helfman and Bada used this information to study age estimation by comparing D/L aspartic acid dental ratios in 20 subjects with good results (r = 0.979). A high coronary D/L ratio was noted in the younger age group, decreasing with age presumptively due to environmental changes. The tooth sectioning was transverse in the Helfman and aspartic acid dental ratios in 20 subjects with good results (r = 0.979). A high coronary D/L ratio was noted in the younger age group, decreasing with age presumptively due to

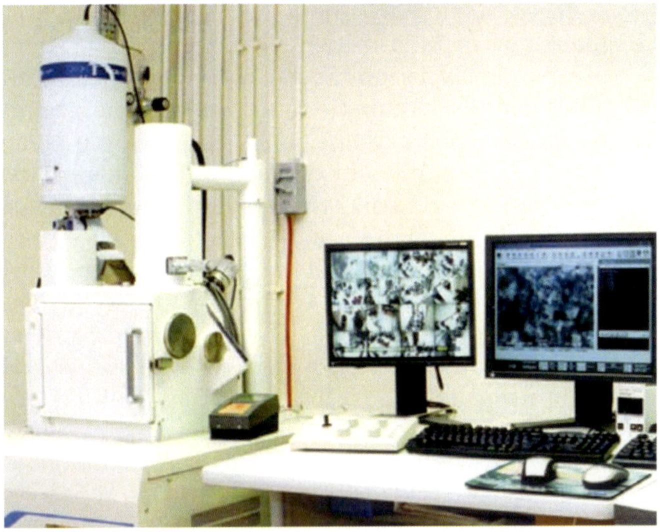

Fig. 11.4

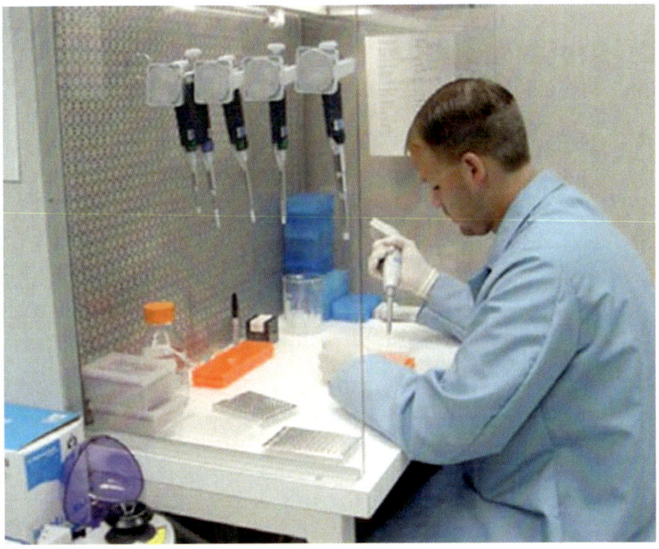

Fig. 11.5

environmental changes. The tooth sectioning was transverse in the Helfman and Bada study. Ogino et al reported this application in forensic odontology specimens for age determination at the time of death. In 1990, Ritz et al reported on the extent of aspartic acid racemization of dentin for age determination at the time of death, concluding that this methodology could provide a more accurate determination of age than other aging parameters. In 1991, Ohtani and Yamamoto studied this aspartic acid relationship using longitudinal sections, with better results (r = 0.991). The teeth used in this study were the lower central incisors and first premolars. Better age estimations could be achieved with fractionating the total amino acid fraction (TAA) into an insoluble collagen fraction (IC) and a soluble peptide fraction, the soluble peptide fraction had higher concentrations of aspartic acid and glutamine, both hydrophilic acids. The technique requires longitudinal sectioning of the tooth and removal of the dental pulp, washing with 0.2 M hydrochloric acid, distilled water, ethanol, and ether (5 min each) and then powdering in an agate mortar. Fractionation and extraction was accomplished by adding 1 ml of 1 M HC1 to 10mg of powder and then centrifuge at 5000 rpm for 1 hr at 5°C. The ratios were then quantitated by gas chromatography using N-trifluoroacetyl isopropyl ester derivatives and a helium carrier gas. These studies yielded age estimations within three to four years of actual age.

- Dental histology has been used for age estimations as well, largely based on the work of Gustafson. Maples in 1978 reported on an improved technique of using dental histology for estimation of adult age by using multiple regression analyses based on Gustafson's parameters of attrition, paradontosis, secondary dentin, cementum, root resorption, and root transparency. He concluded that multiple regression analyses allowed improvement of age estimation in adult human teeth with more precision and less variables. He also noted that the second molar was the best to use for histological aging techniques and that dental aging can be used in the same way as epiphyseal fusion, osteon aging, cranial sutures, and changes in the pulic symphysis have been used in contemporary and prehistoric populations for aging purposes.
- Lipsinic et al studied the correlation of age and incremental lines in the cementum of human teeth and found that direct predictions of age based on these lines generally underestimated the age of older specimens. There was, however, correlation between the number of lines and age.
- Age can be estimated by histological evaluation of osteons in bones. In 1978, Kerley and Ubelaker published a revised method based on the same technique. Both involve use of ground sections and osteon counts. This technique is in common use in anthropology laboratories. Combining bone section histology with dental histology provides a valuable comparative age determination in unknown remains.
- Scanning electron microscopy with and without energy dispersive X-ray analysis has been used to identify teeth by dentinal tubules and evidence of previous restorations especially in incinerated remains.

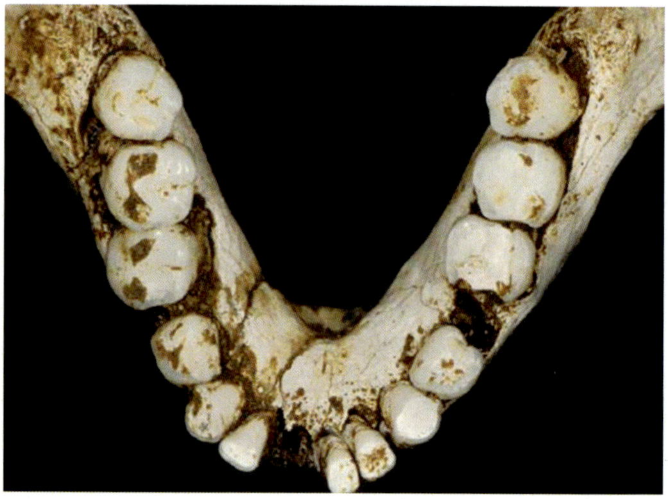

Fig. 11.6

- Carr et al in 1986 reported a case in which the scanning electron microscope was used to confirm dentition in recovered remains from the burned wreckage of a gasoline truck involved in a transportation mishap. Recovered tooth fragments were carbonized and not morphologically recognized as teeth. The desiccated specimens were mounted on aluminum stubs using silver paint, coated with gold-palladium in a sputter-coater, and viewed and photographed on a Joel T-300 SEM at an accelerating voltage of 20 kV. Identification of the specimens as dentition was based on the presence of dentinal tubules. The investigators noted that in addition to dentinal tubules, SEM provided evidence of tool marks and other defects. Use of SEM with EDX provided a profile of elements present which may identify a particular type of dental material. Fairgrieve in 1994 reported a similar case involving SEM on incinerated teeth to evaluate parallel striations in tooth enamel and dentine as evidence of previous dental restorations.

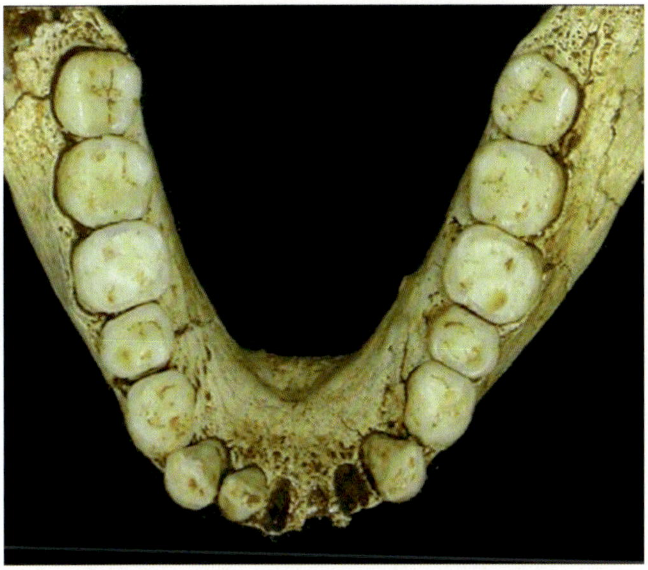

Fig. 11.7

- Smith in 1990 reported the application of SEM with EDS (energy-dispersive X-ray fluorescence spectrometry) analysis of proximal facets. The author concluded that this technique had potential for detecting residual restorative materials in facet areas and in determining the existence and composition of unrecovered adjacent restorations. Smith also noted that this preliminary study indicated that it was possible to detect restorative material residue on the proximal surfaces of unrestored teeth and indicate the antemortem existence of a restoration on the adjacent tooth surface. This knowledge could be valuable in presumptive identifications where the teeth with critical restorations were not recovered with the primary remains, but teeth proximal to those with restorations were present.

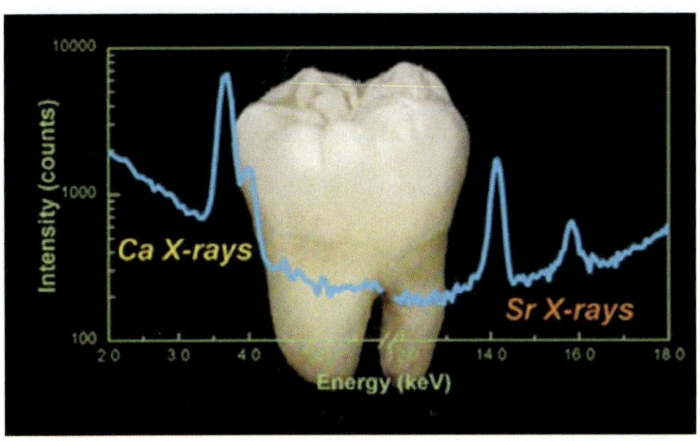

Fig. 11.8

Sorting by Metal Ratios

In 1986, Fulton et al reported on the use of metal ratios in the reassociation of scattered and mixed human bones. This work, conducted at Kansas State University, relied on published work on trace elements present in bone in archaeological materials, especially the work of Lambert et al., who attempted to relate bone metal ratios with diet. Concentrations of 21 elements sampled at 54 places in 30 human bones in each of 5 human skeletons indicated that there were sufficiently consistent metal ratios in bone specimens within an individual to reassociate fragmented remains yet they varied with sufficient discrimination from other individuals to be a useful sorting tool. The magnesium/zinc ratio was the most reliable, with zinc/sodium, magnesium/sodium and chromium/sodium ratios individual trace elements such as arsenic complement this sorting process effort. This ancillary procedure did not provide sufficient individuality to be used alone, but was a valuable adjunct to standard anthropological techniques typically used for sorting commingled remains.

Serological Parameters

- Forensic serology has been applied to odontological investigations with reasonable success. In dental pulps, ABO blood groups and serum proteins Gm, Km, and Gc are present as well as eight polymorphic enzymes (PGM, PGD, ADA, AK, EsD, Fuc, DiA3, and transferrin).
- Kido et al in 1993 reported on the use of transferring C subtyping by isoelectric focusing electrophoresis in dental pulps. Sensitive immunoblotting techniques had previously identified transferring subtypes in urine, blood stains and semen. The Kido et al study showed good correlation between serum and dental pulp specimens.
- Although DNA studies are replacing many of the serological techniques applied to identification efforts, these techniques provide useful sorting data in relatively short periods. Serology continues to play an important role in reassociation efforts in mass disasters, transportation mishaps and explosions when DNA analysis is not readily available or involves a lengthy delay, often up to several months. Serology studies are especially useful when joined with anthropological and odontological methodologies. To get access to the dental pulp, if this is the primary source of the serological material, the tooth must be crushed or sectioned. Many of the techniques used have their basis in similar studies on bone specimens.

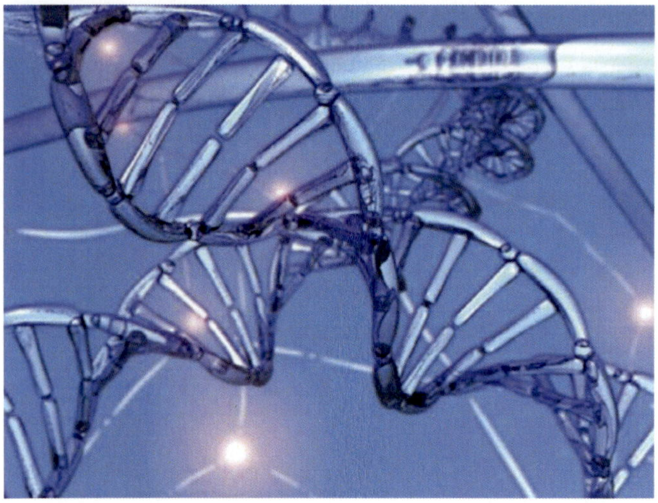

Fig. 11.9

- Lee at el in a series of articles reported on their successes in determining genetic markers in human bone including ABO and IGH grouping using a combination of absorption-elution and two–dimensional absorption-inhibition methodologies. In these studies, bone was cleaned, powdered, then extracted with PBS (phosphate buffered saline) at pH 7.2. They found that the combination of methodologies was more successful than either technique alone.
- Like dental histology techniques for aging, combination of dental and bone serological studies would prove complementary if needed, especially in reassociations. DNA profiling methodologies, like restriction fragment length polymorphism (RFLP) analysis offer similar opportunities but because of DNA degradation often require PCR (polymerase chain reaction) analysis for amplification of allele-specific areas and subsequent study.

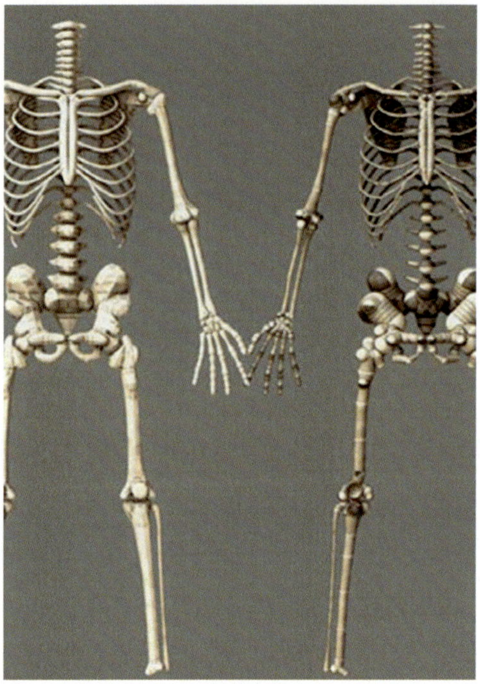

Fig. 11.10

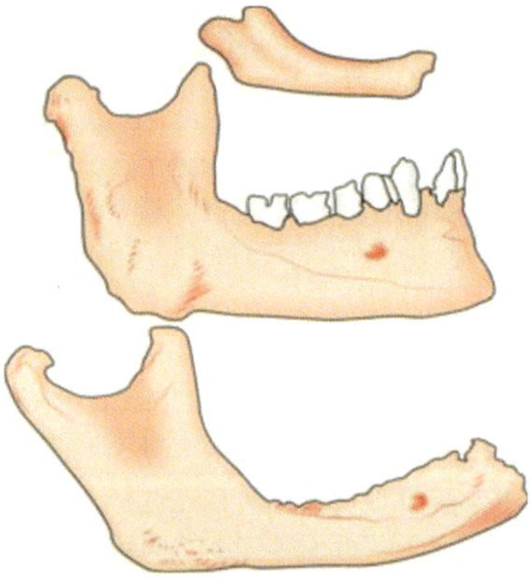

Fig. 11.11

Odontoanthropology

- Ageing methodologies appear equally shared among forensic odontologists, anthropologists, pathologists, and often radiologists. Both anthropologists and radiologists rely heavily on radiographic evidence of aging, dental eruption patterns, and changes in the facial structures with age such as the angle of the mandible, zygomatic arches, and lateral pterygoid plates. Harris and McKee in 1990, studied tooth mineralization characteristic in blacks and whites from the southern US in individuals ranging age from 3.5 to 13 years. They found that females develop more rapidly than males, and that blacks are nearly twice as sexually dimorphic (7.2%) as whites (3.7%). Within each sex, blacks achieved mineralization stages

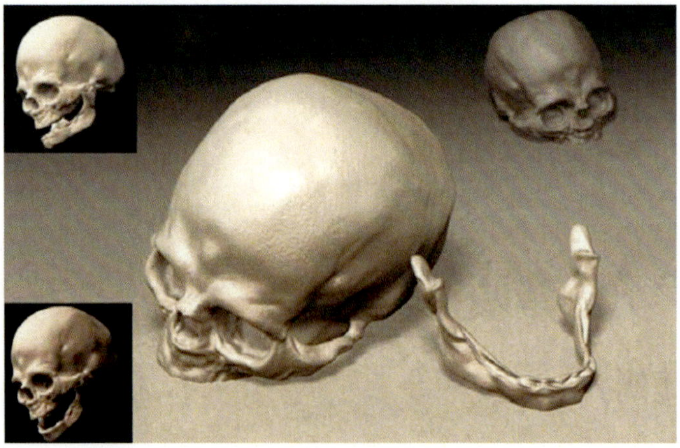

Fig. 11.12

significantly earlier, by approximately 5%, than whites. Many authors do use the human dentition for determinations of age, sex, race, and individualization. He focused on several useful categories; (i) heredity – size and genetic peculiarities, (ii) wear characteristics, (iii) pathology—caries and periodontitis, and (iv) restorations—dental fillings and prostheses such as crowns, bridges, and dentures.

- In 1976, Burns and Maples reported on three parameters of dental aging: Formative, degenerative, and histological. The formative parameter includes tooth mineralization, crown completion, eruption of the crown, and complementary roots. Degenerative measurements include tooth wear, tooth color, and periodontal attachments. Histological assessments include the degree of secondary dentin deposition, cementum apposition, root resorption, and root transparency. The histological measurements and grading follow Gustafson's efforts. Taylor, in studying variations in dental patterns, suggested six parameters for evaluation.
- Type of tooth structure—family characteristics Personal characteristics found throughout a dentition —crowns, occlusal ridges, cusps, and root robusticity, as well as branching patterns, furcation, and fusion,
- Imposed characteristics based on the anatomical relationships of the crowns and roots
- Complexity factors such as tubercles, pits, additional ridges, grooves and fissures
- Acquired characteristics resulting from differences during tooth formation such as hypoplasia, pathology, trauma, function, personal habits, and restorations
- Ethnic considerations.

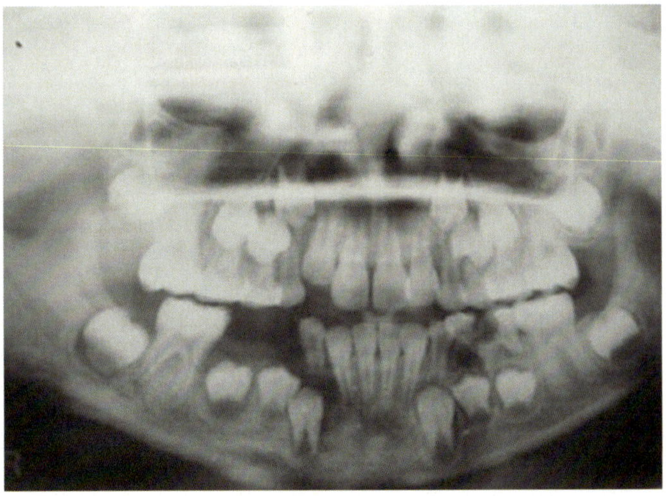

Fig. 11.13

Sex Determinants

Sex determination based on dentition is difficult for most forensic investigators. Sex differences in dentition are based largely on tooth size and shape. Male teeth are usually larger, whereas female canines are more pointed and a narrower buccolingual width. There also appear to be greater differences in size between maxillary central and lateral incisors in females as compared to males. Side-stepping metric differences, Seno and Ishizu reported in 1973 on the use of the Y chromosome in dental pulp to determine sex differences. Success in sexing unknown remains based on this technique have resulted in several published accounts. Studies involved the detection of the Y chromosome using quinacrine and fluorescent microscopy. This microscopic approach to sexing would appear more reliable to the forensic odontologist than metrics, at least on difficult, incomplete remains. The successful isolation of sex-specific banding patterns in DNA profiles of the X and Y chromosomes developed from fresh and degraded specimens.

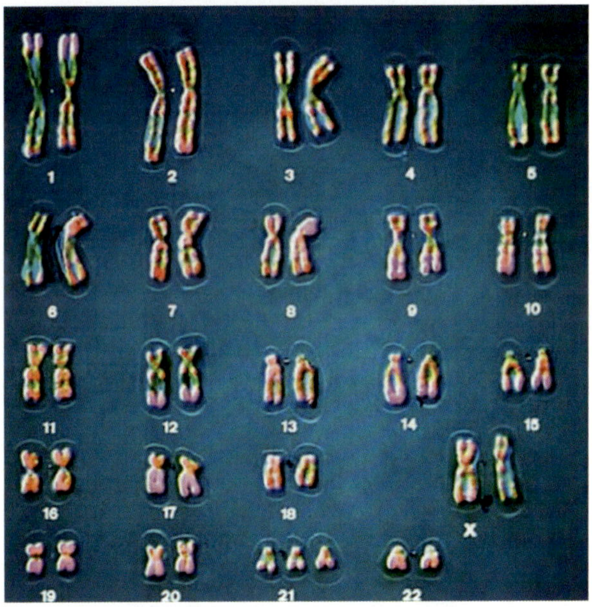

Fig. 11.14

Racial Determinants

- Race determination in skeletal remains traditionally focuses on craniofacial characteristics such as the proportions of the orbital and nasal areas, nasal aperture characteristics, lower nasal border features, lower facial prognathism, palate form, cheekbone contours and incisors shoveling. For each of the osteological clues, they pointed out the need to consider.

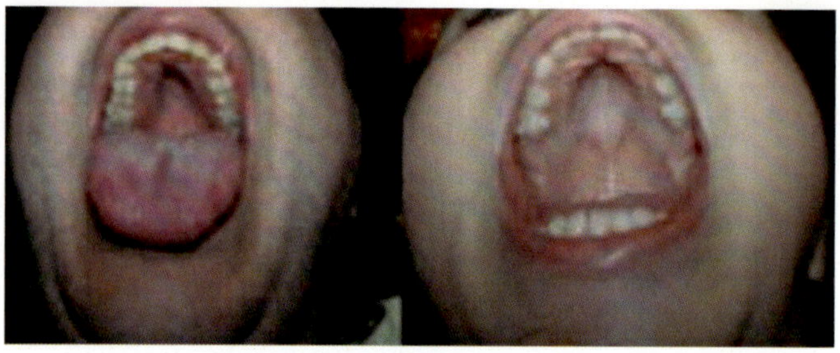

Fig. 11.15

- Its basic etiology : Whether it is primarily biochemical, hormonal, or activity-related in order to predict its variation pattern.
- Its range of variation by sex in various racial/ethnic groups

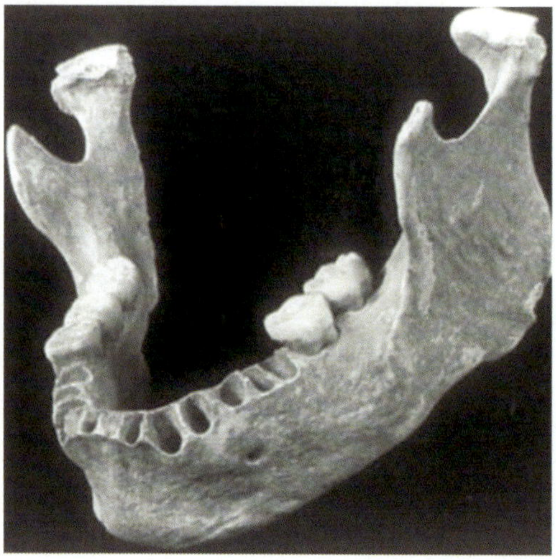

Fig. 11.16

- Its manifestation by age: The age at which it appears and its pattern of change from childhood to old age,
- How it is influenced by health, nutrition, occupation, or other circumstances of an individual's life
- Whether there are secular changes in its expression
- Whether the characteristics are real, but temporary.

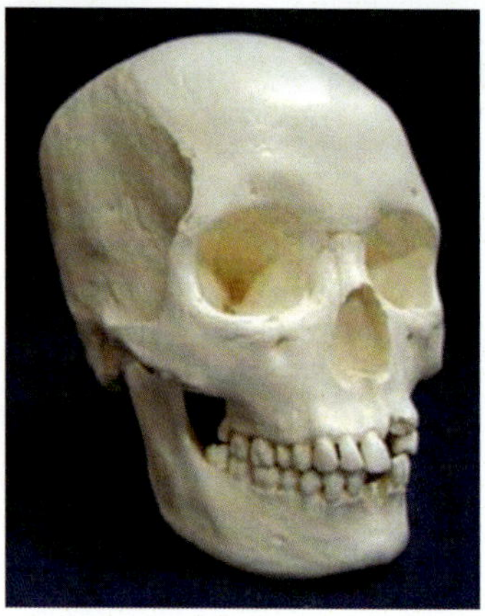

Fig. 11.17

- From a dental perspective, both the mandible and dentition reflect racial characteristics. Projecting chins are found in Europeans and some Asiatics. Rounded, almost receding, chins are found in Australian aborigines and in some South Pacific Islanders. Most African and Afro-American chins are intermediate. General jaw-shaped corresponds with general skull-shaped. Whereas large bizygomatic widths with wide mandibles have deep rami and significant gonial flare. The greatest eversion is found in Eskimos and Amer-Indians. Rocker jaws seem associated with Hawaiian crania. These general characteristics reflect relative ethnic dental markers.

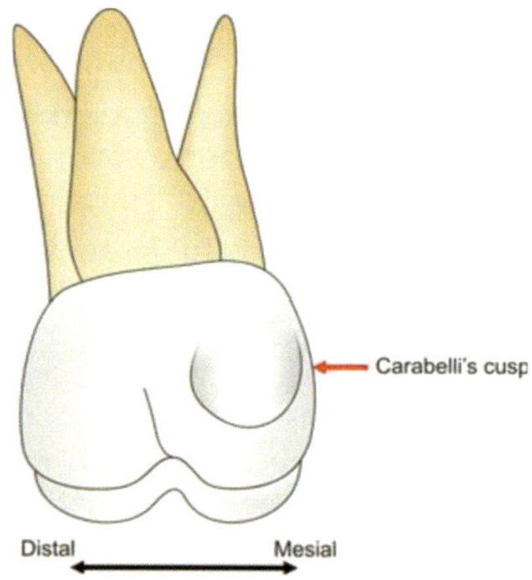

Fig. 11.18

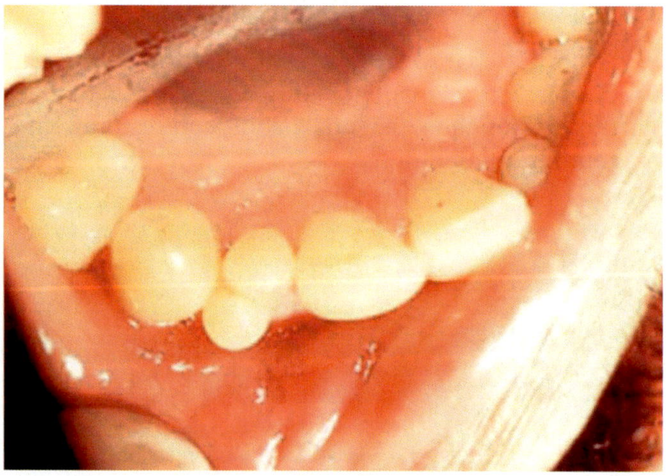

Fig. 11.19

- According to these authors, the most useful racial clue in dentition is "shovel-shaped" incisors found in most Asiatic Mongoloids and Amerindians and in less than 10% of whites and blacks. Tooth size and shape including shovel tooth incisors, Carabelli's cusp or tubercle, enamel pearls, and dental pulp shape (taurodontism vs cynodontism) have been listed as racial determinants.

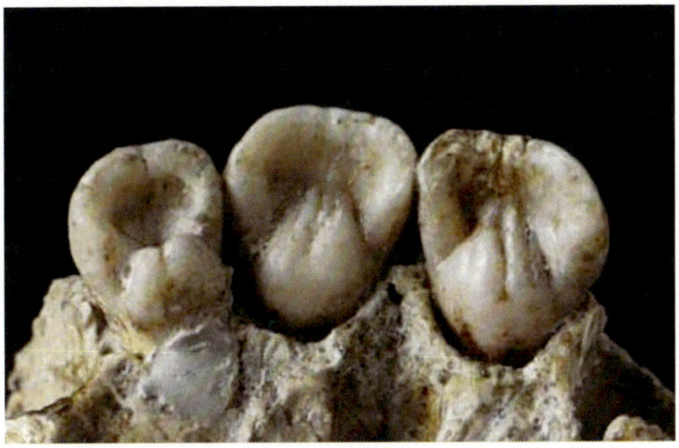

Fig. 11.20

- Carabelli's tubercle or cusp is an anomalous cuspule on the mesiolingual surface of maxillary incisors appearing in 50% of American whites, 34% of Afro-Americans, and 5 to 20% of Ameindians. Taurodontism or "bulltoothness", especially in maxillary molars, enamel pearls on premolars, and the frequent congenital lack of upper third molars, are commonly noted features in Mongoloids.

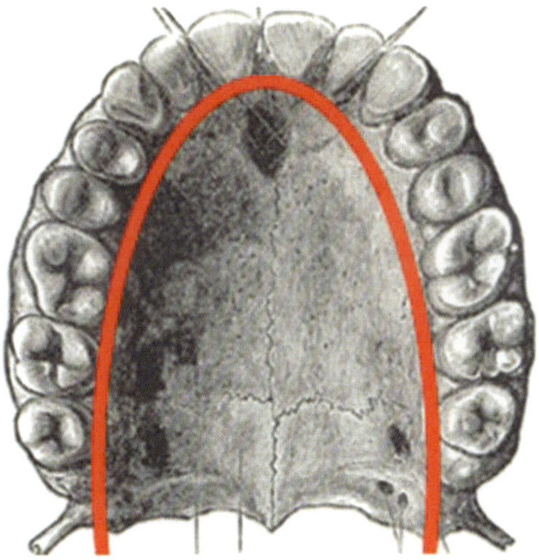

Fig. 11.21

- The form and shape of the dental arches are subject to considerable variation. Stewart in described these forms as ovoid, U-shaped, and horseshoe-snape. Martin and Saller in 1956 described these forms as semicircular, half ellipse, paraboloid, and broken angular line. The proportion of the palate and the associated dental arches are indicated by the palatal index, the ratio of the width to the length of the palate.
- There are large-toothed and small-toothed races. Aboriginal Australians, the Melanesians, and the American Indian including the Eskimos tend to be large-toothed, with wide crowns. The Lapps and Bushmen are small people with small teeth. American blacks tend to have large crowns.
- Skull measurements have been used by many examiners as a basis for racial determinations. In South America, the Bonwill triangle, an equilateral mandibular triangle connecting the apex of the mesial contact areas of the two central mandibular central incisors with the two mandibular condyles, has been used on the assumption that the studied population groups are not mixed and retain consistent hereditary characteristics.
- Removal, modification, or decoration of anterior teeth can be useful indicators of sex or race. These cultural characteristics often reflect geographic ethnic patterns.
- These craniofacial and dental issues take on some relevance when efforts are made to reconstruct likely ages based on skeletal craniofacial characteristics. Caldwell described four current methods of facial

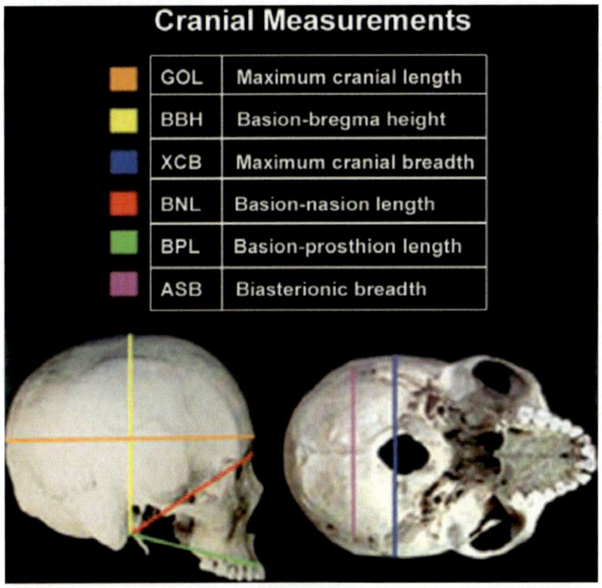

Fig. 11.22

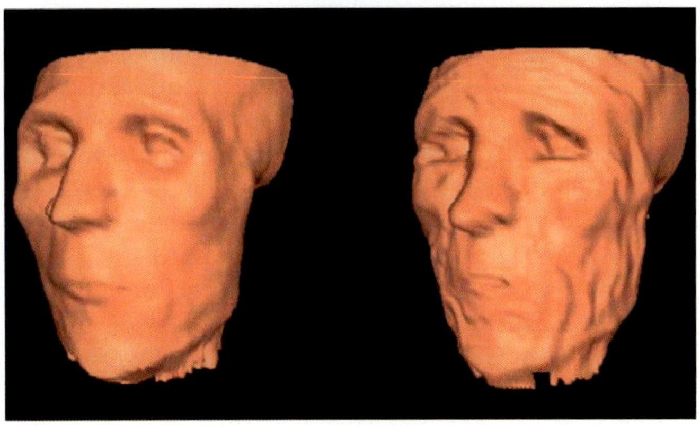

Fig. 11.23

reconstruction: (i) Modeling in clay directly on the skull (three-dimensional), (ii) Construction of artists' drawings (two dimensional), (iii) Restoration of disrupted or damaged tissues, and (iv) Photographic or portrait superimpositions.

- Webster et al reported on the identification of human remains using photographic reconstructions in two methods, comparative and superimpositions. This report used photographs, potraits, and dental studies to confirm the identifications.
- Rathbun et al emphasized the eyes, lips, nasal form, and hair style as the most significant facial features in recognition. Lenorovitz and Sussman listed skin, hair, skin color, ears, face shape, eyebrows, eyes, nose, lips, eye color, chin age, and cheeks in order of importance to visual recognition. Computerized techniques such as computer age progression studies which have proven to be a valuable identification technique in missing persons investigations. Fierro discussed this technique in a comprehensive review of human identification problems in unknown decedents and the variety of techniques used to resolve these problems.

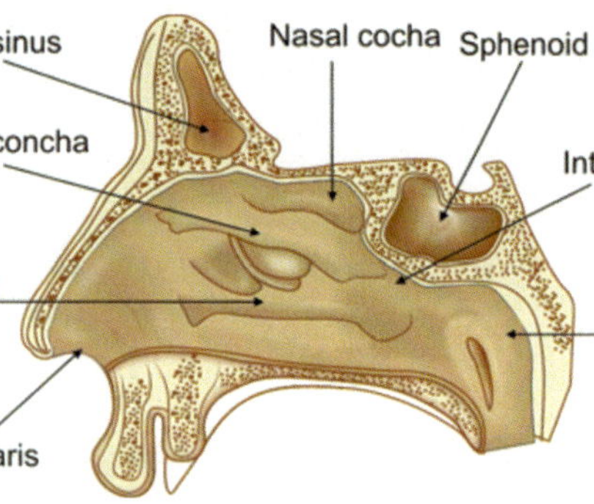

Fig. 11.24

FORENSIC ODONTOLOGICAL DATABASES

Applications in Mass Disasters

- The Department of Defense uses two important databases in its forensic odontological identification efforts: (i) A pantomorphograph registry which is periodically updated by copies of pantomorphographs in each servicemember's dental record, and (ii) Widespread use of a temporary computerized identification sorting tool known as CAPMI (Computerized Assisted Postmortem Identification System) restoration identification and comparison showed a high degree of specificity. Several other dental computer sorting systems have been developed and are in beta testing. Current interest in the digitalization of radiographs for teleradiology and

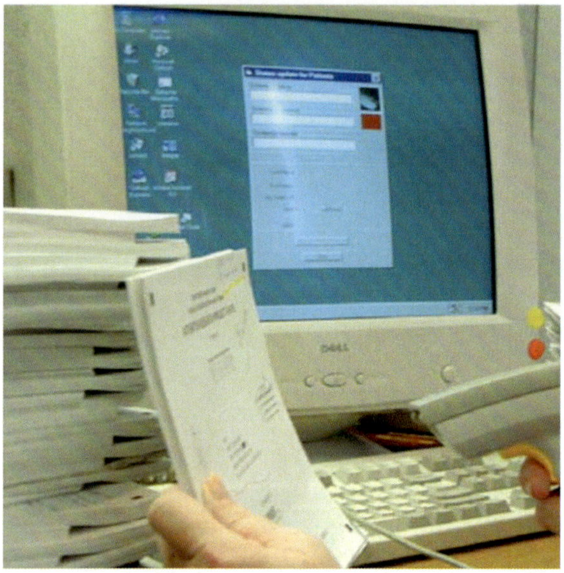

Fig. 11.25

telemedicine purposes and its potential application to dental radiographs such as pantomorphographs, especially in established databank, should improve such dental databases and provide an important tool in decedent identification efforts. This digitalized image retrieved from a databank could be compared with actual pantomorphographs and apical films in the victim's dental record as a validation means of premortem identification and then compared with postmortem dental records developed during the investigation. This DNA material is not routinely typed, but rather stored in the registry under stringent environmental controls for possible use in the event of the servicemember's death in operational missions.

- There has been considerable debate on the applications of such databanks relative to an individual's constitutional rights of privacy and freedom from self-incrimination. This concern has been especially applied to proposed or existent DNA databanks. Databanks that provide the population genetic studies so critical to the inter-pretation of DNA typing results relative to a specific identification.

Bitemark Examinations

- Bitemark examinations relative to scientific evidence and the potential use of ancillary technologies to resolve certain identification issues. A review of the published literature on bitemarks underscores the significance in specimen examination and evaluation with any obtained templates or known impressions relative to: (i) The relationship of the jaws, (ii) The form and size of arches (iii) Missing teeth, (iv) Spacing between teeth (v) Presence of supernumerary teeth

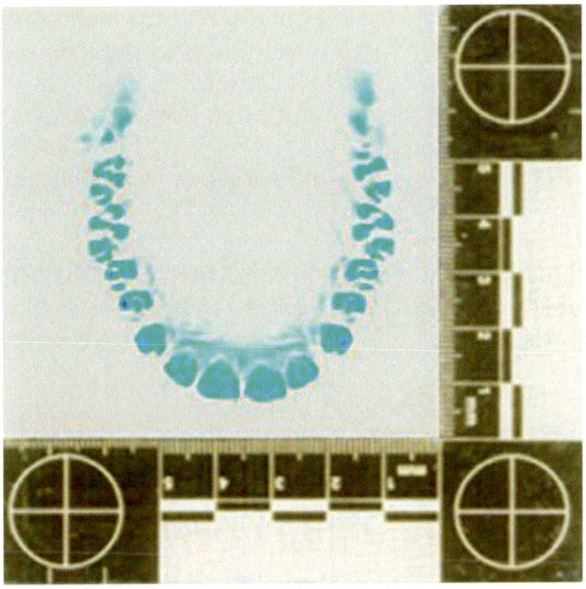

Fig. 11.26

(vi) Observed rotations of teeth (vii) The width of teeth, and (viii) Presence of special features such as fractures and ridges. Discussions focus on the identification of bitemarks, their documentation photographically, and the level of individualization possible based on the documented and preserved evidence against templates of dentition of individuals under investigation in the case. The use of fingerprint powder or fingerprint ink on bitemark impressions to enhance impression visibility. Soft tissue radiography has also been used to enhance bitemark impressions.

- Legal challenges to bitemark evidence seems to fall into two major categories of admissibility : (i) Reliability of analysis, and (ii) Violations of constitutional rights (Fourth and Fifth Amendments) regarding search and seizure and self-incrimination protections.
- One aspect of bitemark investigations often neglected is the role of ancillary chemical and serological studies which either support the identification of the observed injury as a bitemark or the specificity of the bitemark relative to the biter's sex, race, or individuality. One such series of study focused on the presence of saliva and its serological characteristics. Another parameter, often mentioned, is the potential use of cytological examinations of exfoliated buccal epithelial cells, especially for sex determination and/or DNA analysis.
- Saliva offers several routes of inquiry. Its identification in bitemarks is directed towards the identification of inorganic anions such as thiocyanate or nitrites and polymorphic enzymes such as alkaline phosphatase and amylase. Further individualization, if pursued, is directed towards classical serological parameters including the detection of blood groups, serum polymorphic enzymes, and polymorphic studies unique to saliva based on electrophoretic variation of isoenzymes of hexose-6-phosphate dehydrogenase (Sgd), amylase, acid protein (Pa), basic protein (Pb), double band protein (Db), and proline rich protein (Pr).

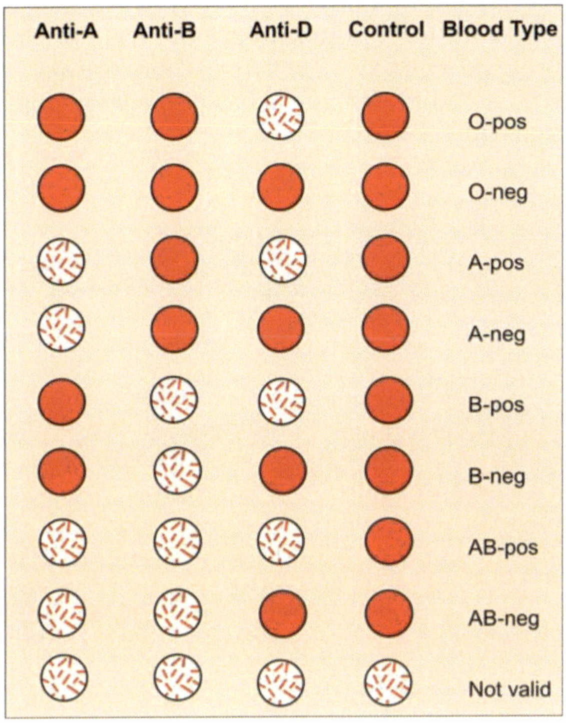

Fig. 11.27

Chemical Markers

- The detection of the thiocyanate ion (3.1 to 27.5 mg SCN/100 ml) in saliva relies on the calorimetric reaction of thiocyanate with dilute ferric chloride to the slightly acidified specimen producing a pink to red product which is sensitive to 3 µg SCN. Thiocyanate in saliva persists for some time and has been reported present, although reduced, 28 months after deposition. A negative test for thiocyanate does not exclude the presence of saliva in a stain. When present in fresh samples, the average is 9.3 mg/100 mL and is about 2.5 times higher in smokers than nonsmokers.
- Nitrite exists in saliva in concentrations of 4.6 to 10 µg NO_2/ml and is detected using the Griess test which using sulfanilic acid forms a diazonium compound which reacts with naphthylamine to form a diazonium compound which reacts with naphthylamine compound. The test is sensitive but less specific for saliva and is limited to use in recent depositions.

A reagent consisting of 0.5% alpha-naphthylamine in 5N acetic acid and 0.8% sulfanilic acid in 5N acetic acid was used in the salivary stain studies.

- A very sensitive and relatively specific general test for saliva is the demonstration of significant amounts of amylase in a suspect stain. A number of technologies have been described but those most used in forensic investigations utilize starch dye substrates using Renazol Blue R, Cibachrom blue F3G, or Procion Brillant Red M2BS. Positive reactions are also noted with ascorbic acid which has also been reported in saliva in 2.4 to 4.6 µg/ml concentrations.

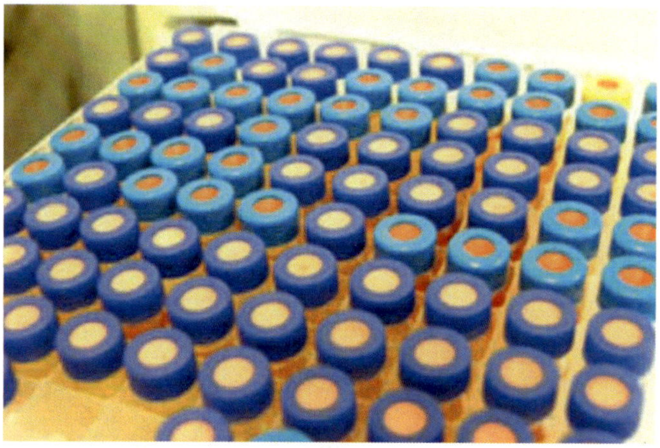

Fig. 11.28

Serological Markers

- General serological parameters used for identification purposes rely on the presence and detection of blood groups in biological specimens other than blood detectable in 80% of the population based on secretor status. In addition to the ABH, Lewis, and Sda antigens, a number of serum polymorphic isoenzymes are present in saliva: alkaline phosphatase, amylase, esterases, G-6-PD, and parotid peroxidase (SAPX).

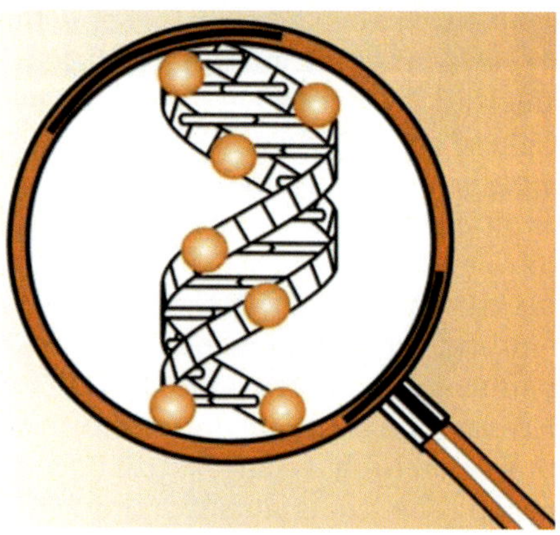

Fig. 11.29

Saliva also contains an interesting polymorphic protein system based on parotid glycoproteins; most if not all are acidic and proline rich. Both Gm and Km proteins are present and have been used for racial determinations.

- Typical serological studies of saliva are usually limited to detection of amylase, ABH, and Lewis antigens and several polymorphic markers. DNA profiling offers other possibilities, including greater individualization, if enough DNA can be extracted from any exfoliated cells.

Salivary Drug Detection

- The use of saliva in drug detection has been explored, especially in monitoring therapeutic drug concentrations study which found measurable quantities of drugs in saliva extracted with methanol and analyzed by EMIT (enzyme multiple immuno-assay technique) and gas chromatography/mass spectrophotometry. This methodology, both specific and sensitive appears to be a useful adjunct to serological testing in bitemarks for identification purposes. A number of drugs such as phenobarbital, amphetamine and morphine have been detected in saliva and saliva stains by radioimmunoassay (RIA) by a number of investigators.
- Fletcher et al in 1984 described an ELISA (enzyme-linked immunoassay) technique using monoclonal antibody based on the presence of salivary IgA for species identification in stains up to 16 months old. Cross reactivity was limited and readily identifiable. Crossover electrophoresis and double gel diffusion techniques were used for comparison in cases with poor monoclonal antibody results. This technique would appear to have value in bitemark examinations from nonhumans where the biting animal is not known.

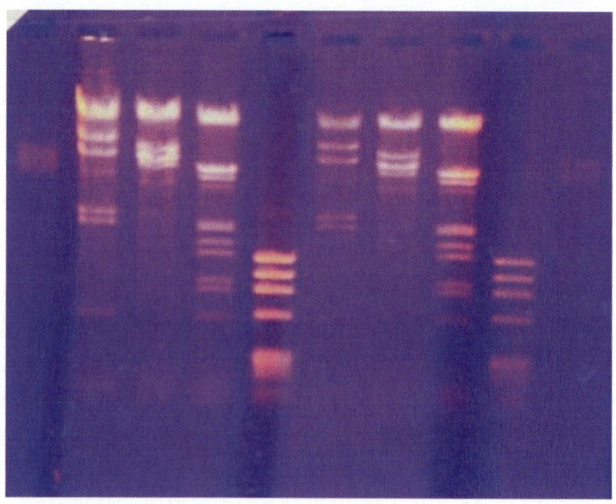

Fig. 11.30

- Sensabaugh and Blake, in a review of DNA analysis using polymerase chain reaction (PCR) applications, commented on its use in species determinations. Evolutionary relationships among species are most directly determined by comparisons at the DNA sequence level. For routine species determination, simple yes/no amplication assays for species-specific sequences can be utilized. Alternatively, amplification coupled with dot blot hybridization with species-specific probes can be used. If an unknown cannot be directly identified by sequencing, it can be placed into a genus, family, or order by comparing its sequence to corresponding sequences from other species groups. The sequence region for which most comparative sequence data exist is the cytochrome β gene on mitochondrial DNA. The gene has conservative sequence regions that allow the design of "universal" primers that will amplify the gene in most vertebrate species.

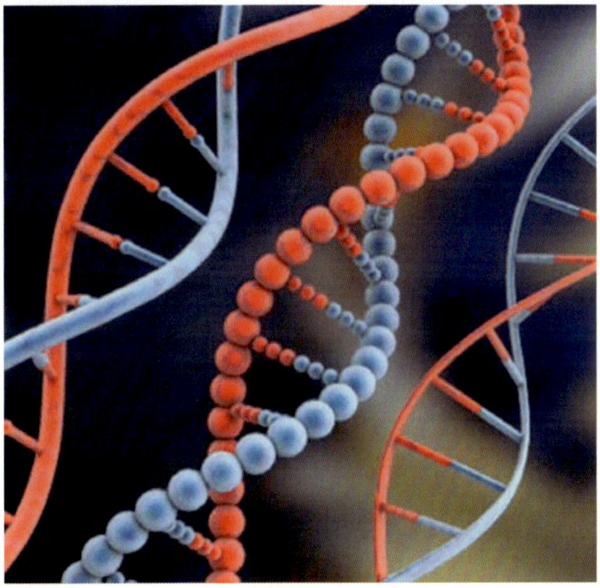

Fig. 11.31

Sex Determination in Bitemarks

- The possibility of obtaining exfoliated buccal epithelial cells in saliva on bitemarks has increased the possibility of sex determination of the perpetrator. The duration of this line of inquiry is apparently possible for several weeks postdepositions, depending on the materials containing the impressions and environmental factors. Two parameters have been proposed, both based on successful efforts to sex bloodstains: (i) The presence and detection of sex chromatin (Barr bodies in females, and F bodies in males); and (ii) Sex hormone level determinations based on detectable quantities and ratios of testosterone and 17B-estradiol by radioimmunoassay (RIA). The former parameter has been demonstrated successfully in saliva stains.
- Interpretation of such investigatory efforts must be dependent on an understanding of the possible variations that might be encountered. Discrepancies noted in tests for sex chromatin include: (i) Chromatin negative females, e.g. Turner's Syndrome and testicular feminization, (ii) Chromatin positive males, e.g., Klinefelter's Syndrome, and (iii) Genetic mosaics. In each case, a sufficient number of nucleated class must be obtained, fixed, and stained. Alcohol fixation and H&E stains have been used successfully for detection of Barr bodies or "drumsticks" in materials containing at least 100 nucleated cells. An aceto-orcein staining process was described by Sanderson and Stewart in 1961.
- Determination of sex by DNA analysis according to Sensabaugh and Blake is possible by using PCR based on the characteristics of the mammalian sex chromosomes, X and Y. Normal females have two X chromosomes and males have an X and Y chromosome. The development of a mammalian embryo as male is determined by genes on the Y chromosome and the phenotypic sex of individuals with an abnormal complement of sex chromosomes depends only on the presence or absence of the Y chromosome. Several PCR-based approaches have been used. The simplest is the amplication of a Y specific sequence; the presence of a PCR product indicates the sample contains male cells. With this assay, the absence of a product cannot be interpreted unless there is an amplication control. An assay using the DYZI repeat sequence for the Y marker and either an Alu repeat or DQA sequences as amplication controls is an example of such testing.
- Male DNA shows both X and Y PCR products, whereas female DNA shows only the X product. A third method,

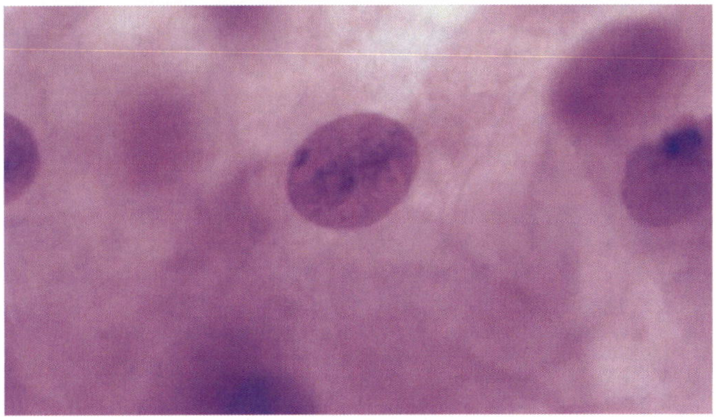

Fig. 11.32

described by Aasen and Medrano amplifies both the X and Y specific sequences using a single primer set. The human ZFY and ZFX genes possess regions of conserved sequence permitting the design of primers capable of amplifying both.

DNA Analysis in Biological Specimens

- DNA analysis has provided a significant advance in identification efforts and is routinely used in criminal investigations and mass disasters. The relative absence of general population DNA identification databanks against which putative specimens can be compared complicates identification of the decedent. If a presumptive identification is available, however, then it is often possible by using either nuclear or mitochondrial DNA profiling analysis to confirm the identification of the unknown and to reassociate remains when other methodologies are not applicable. In mass disasters, a common approach is to identify fragmentary remains by traditional means such as dental comparisons, fingerprints, or radiographic criteria (superimpositions), type recovered DNA from these fragments, and use that profile to reassociate other fragmentary remains producing the same DNA profile pattern. Current DNA profiling or fingerprinting techniques are either restriction fragment length polymorphisms (RFLPs) on variable number tandem repeats (VNTRs) or polymerase chain reaction (PCR) analysis. The PCR technique or allele-specific analysis focuses in on and amplifies a specific DNA region. Differences among individuals at that site can be distinguished through the use of specialized probes that trigger a color change or through gel electrophoresis followed by a silver stain. Forensic PCR methods cannot discriminate among individuals as well as RFLP analysis does, but PCR requires only small amounts of DNA (approximately 1% that required for RFLP analysis) and can be used with some degraded DNA.

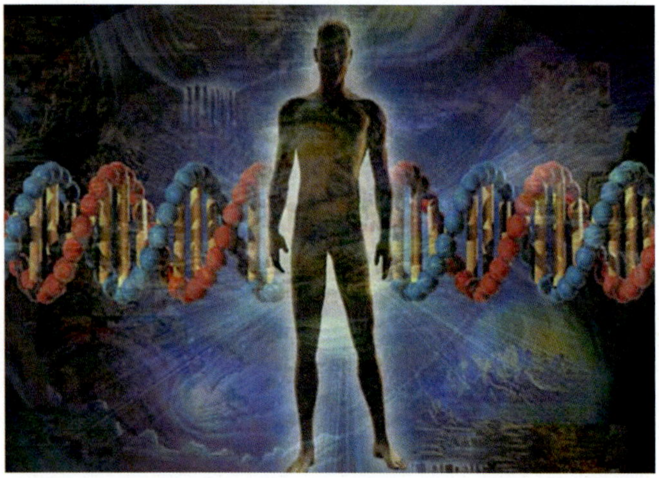

Fig. 11.33

- Approximately 70 to 80% of the DNA in the total human genome consists of unique sequences including spacer DNA, signal sequences, and protein coding DNA. The remaining 20 to 30% of the genome consists of repetitive, primarily noncoding sequences of uncertain function. It is on these sequences that DNA profiling depends. Repetitive DNA can be divided into two classes: (i) Tandemly repetitive sequences, and (ii) Interspersed repeats. Tandem repetitive DNA accounts for approximately 1/3 of the repetitive DNA (10% of the genome) and is divided into two categories: (i) Satellite DNA, ranging from 5 to 250 base pairs repeated many times, and (ii) Short tandem repeats, much shorter than satellite DNA. Which exhibit a high degree of variability in overall length; these regions are also termed "minisatellites" or VNTRs (variable number tandem repeats) located at unique chromosomal loci. Minisatellites are relatively long tandem repeats whereas shorter repeats fall into the short tandem repeats (STRs) described above consisting of "core sequences". The different DNA profiling techniques focus on one or more of these repetitive sequence areas.

DNA Contamination Issues

- Invariably, such DNA analysis using RFLP or PCR techniques raise concerns of contamination and subsequently reliability in interpretation of so-called matches. A number of studies have addressed these issues, especially in regard to the use of RFLP (restriction fragment length polymorphisms) methodology.
- Adams et al in 1991 reported on investigations conducted by the FBI relative to this issue based on profile results obtained from bloodstains and other biological stains subjected to a mixture of other biological stains, environmental insults (sunlight and temperature), different substrates (cotton, nylon, blue denim, glass, aluminum, and wood), and contaminants including gasoline, bleach, sodium hydroxide, soil, motor oil, detergent, phosphate salt, glacial acetic acid, and microorganisms. They found that in those samples which did produce profiles, those profiles were consistent with those of untreated control samples.
- In 1993, Webb et al revisited this issue using microbial challenges of variable number tandem repeats (VNTR) probes for DNA profiling. Numerous polymorphic

markers cloned from variable number tandem repeat sequences have been described and used for individual identification purposes. These clones usually consist of several kilobases of VNTR sequence suitable for isototopic labeling Recently, however, synthetic oligonucleotides complementary to VNTRs have been used as DNA probes. Reporter molecules including biotin, digoxigenin, and alkaline phosphatase are covalently linked to the oligonucleotides facilitating nonisotopic detection methods. This study used probes challenged with DNA isolated from a variety of bacterial, yeast, and fungal sources. No DNA sequences of nonhuman origin were visualized on either autoradiographs or lumigraphs. High molecular weight DNA can be obtained when blood and semen stains are subjected to environmental and contaminating factors.

DNA Dental Applications

- Schwartz et al reported a interesting study of DNA obtained from teeth subjected to a variety of environmental conditions. The studies were on dental pulp using restriction enzyme digestion with PstI and restriction fragment length polymorphisms on loci DZS44, DXYS14, D18S27, and DXZ1. The authors obtained good results but observed band shifting of 2 to 4 kilobases with increased temperatures. This technical artifact can make pattern or band interpretation difficult in potential matches.
- Smith et al in 1993 reported on a systematic approach to sampling dental DNA for identification purposes. The study was based on crushed and sectioned tooth specimens which were subjected to DNA typing with both sequence—and length-based analyses comparing teeth from the same individual and with other individuals. The authors concluded that crushing specimens maximizes the yield of dental DNA but with greater degradation, and that substantial yields could be obtained from more conservative sectioning efforts. The method of sampling did not affect the ability to do DNA typing. High molecular weight DNA was obtained from all specimens. DNA typing studies were also successfully performed on powdered dentin and dental roots, providing high molecular weight DNA. The dental roots yielded more DNA but it was also more degraded. The mitochondrial DNA control area was amplified for all molar pulp extracts.
- When DNA is highly degraded, or in limited quantities, mitochondrial DNA (mtDNA) can be used for human identification and evidentiary materials. Mitochondrial DNA constitutes a fraction of 1% of the total DNA in a cell. However, there are hundreds to thousands of copies of mtDNA for every copy of nuclear DNA. The maternal inheritance pattern increases the availability of matching sequences of individuals with siblings and even distant maternal cousins who should carry the identical mtDNA sequence. Further use of this technology will be dependent on the establishment of DNA databases and population statistical studies to support interpretation of results.

DNA Profiling or Fingerprinting

- DNA profiling or fingerprinting is based on the fact that although most of the DNA molecule is common to all humans, parts differ from person to person. With the exception of identical siblings, the DNA of every individual is unique. DNA identification tests use sophisticated techniques of molecular biology developed over the last 25 years to compare samples taken from a suspect with those found in blood, semen, hair roots, or cells from saliva or skin discovered at a crime scene. In paternity cases, DNA from the alleged father is compared with that of the mother and child.
- The most useful DNA identification tests currently available analyze highly variable regions of human DNA called restriction fragment length polymorphisms (RFLPs). In this technique, genomic DNA is isolated from the cells nuclei and cut into fragments by a restriction enzyme that cleaves the DNA at specific locations, recognizing only certain combinations of the ATCG codes on the DNA molecule. The sizes of the resulting fragments differ from individual to individual because of polymorphisms, highly variable DNA regions that contain a variable number of repeating units of certain small DNA sequences. The resulting fragments are separated by slab gel electrophoresis into different-sized bands. The DNA is then extracted from the gel when it is blotted onto a nylon membrane using the Southern blotting technique where a series of radioactive variations are common. The probes used are segments of known DNA impregnated with radioactive phosphorus 32 which bind to the precise DNA fragments tested, transferring their radio-activity selectively to those fragments. The membrane is then plaed on X-ray film exposing the film to the radiation in the phosphorus and visualizing the DNA fragment. The process is lengthy, with each of the four or five loci exposed sequentially it usually takes 10 weeks. Once the film is developed it is inspected by the investigator and at least one other expert and often scanned into a computer for precise measurement and comparison of the resulting bands with known samples of DNA. Ambiguity in

interpretation of these bands results from band shifts, degradation, missing bands, extra bands and combined bands, all due to technical problems. The dilemma faced by the analyst is how to distinguish differences induced by technical problems and artifacts from true genetic differences between samples.

- A second type of DNA profiling is polymerase chain reaction (PCR) which is a molecular copying process for developing gene sequences. A typical PCR test looks at six different inherited traits, each controlled by a specific gene, each with two alleles; one maternal allele and one paternal allele. If the alleles are different, the individual is homozygous for that trait. For 6 different genes, there are just 21 possible combinations of alleles: 6 homozygous and 15 heterozygous. PCR looks for matches for these 21 combinations, some of which are extremely rare. The results are recorded as colored dots on a nylon strip. The PCR technique focuses on and amplifies a specific DNA region. The differences among individuals at that site are distinguished through the use of specialized probes which trigger a color change or through gel electrophoresis followed by a silver stain. Forensic PCR methods are less specific than RFLP analysis with probabilities of 1:100 to 1:2000 as compared with 1:10,000 to 1:1,000,000 reported for RFLP. However, PCR requires extremely small quantities of DNA and can be used on degraded specimens. A sizable evidence sample, however, does not guarantee a good yield of analyzable material. Heat, moisture, sunlight, surface contaminants, and other factors can speed DNA degradation. Contamination of evidence with DNA from animals or bacteria is usually not a problem because the probes used in DNA profiling are specific to humans or at least primates. Bacteria does have an effect on the stability of human DNA, especially soil bacteria which are rich in nucleases.
- Criminal cases generate more controversy than paternity suits. Both require a documented chain of evidence, however the forensic material may be limited as compared to samples from paternity cases. It often takes more work to isolate DNA from forensic specimens and more probes and controls. The most disputatious issue of forensic DNA identification efforts involves population genetics. Scientists disagree on how to calculate the probability that a suspect's DNA profile could match the evidence by chance. At issue is a method called the multiplication or product rule which assumes that the tested loci follow the Hardy-Weinberg equilibrium principle of independence. The chance that a suspect's DNA coincidentally matches the evidence depends on how frequently the particular pattern of genetic variants (alleles) present in the DNA profile occurs in the general population.

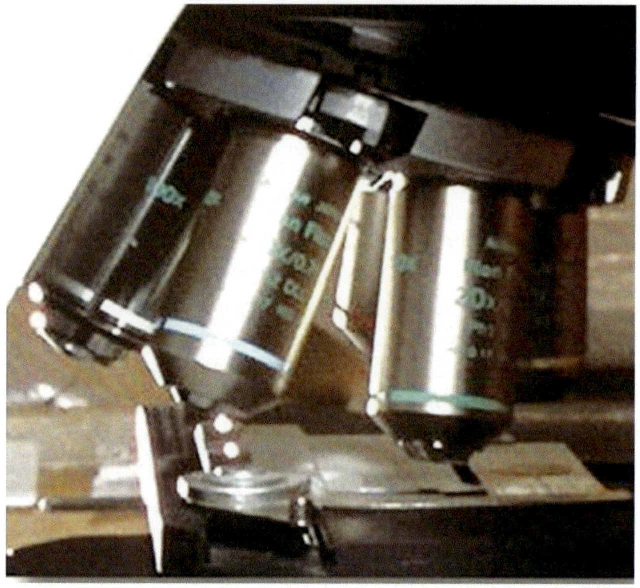

Fig. 11.34

- This issue arises because DNA profiling analyzes only a small sample of an individual's full complement of DNA, some 3 billion base pairs in the human genome. Both profiling methods reduce the possibility of random matches by evaluating more than one specific locus on DNA. In an RFLP analysis employing four or five single locus probes, each probe is designed to recognize a particular locus on a specific chromosome. Forensic laboratories compile databases of the alleles that are found with each employed probe. These individual probes yield frequencies which in the multiplication rule provide a probability of matching patterns by the multiplication of the frequency of each of the used probes. The multiplication rule derives from population genetics models that assume that the DNA variations revealed by each probe are inherited independently of each other.
- The FBI and other forensic laboratories concede that the distribution of alleles is not completely random. These laboratories report the calculated probabilities of a random match for each of these data groups and the frequencies can vary widely. These large pools are not discriminatory enough because there is as much genetic variation amoung subgroups within races as there is between races. They recommended a more conservative approach called the ceiling principle in which forensic scientists would use the highest observed frequency of a given allele or 5%, whichever is larger, to calculate the likelihood of a random match.

The report called for research to set these ceiling frequencies by using empirical data suggesting that determining the actual frequencies of particular DNA variations. Six objections have been raised to the ceiling principle:

(i) The ceiling principle is premised on the flawed analysis of Lewontin and Hartl that there is significant population substructure.
(ii) The ceiling principle is scientifically flawed because it is not used in population genetics; moreover, the plan to sample 10 to 15 representative populations is statistically unsound.
(iii) The ceiling principle makes unwarranted assumptions about the possible substructure of a populations,
(iv) The ceiling principle is so conservative that it hampers the courtroom application of DNA fingerprintings,
(v) The ceiling principle is not actually guaranteed to be conservative, and
(vi) The NRC report is causing DNA fingerprinting cases to be thrown out of court.

- Standardization is also being driven by the creation of the national DNA databank. This system is called CODIS (combined DNA index system) and will enable investigators to compare DNA profiles derived from evidence from rapes or murders with DNA profiles from convicted offenders from throughout the country. They also will be able to compare evidence from unsolved crimes in other jurisdictions and check profiles of missing persons. The national database means that each laboratory must be able to reproducibly generate DNA profiles. The threat of privacy posed by the expanding use of DNA databanks is an increasingly prominent issue according to some legal scholars. Although the DNA regions targeted by current profiling methods do not code for disease or any identifiable physical traits, some observers are disturbed by the government's access to such information.
- Williams et al published a recent article on the analysis of DNA restriction fragments and polymerase chain reaction products by capillary electrophoresis. Lifecodes and other companies have developed chemiluminescent probe systems that can replace the radioactive probes used in RFLP. Currently used in paternity testing, this methodology has forensic interest.
- The application of this DNA technology to forensic odontology cases relies on the principles presented and the general condition that this analysis will be done by other than forensic odontologists. DNA has been isolated and characterized from dental pulp. This success provides a basis for reassociation of body parts that might not be otherwise possible because of decomposition. There is particular interest in mitochondrial DNA analysis because of its availability, especially in skeletal materials and its successful characterization by polymerase chain reaction.

Issues of Scientific Testing: General Principles

- Scientific evidence has special relevance in medicolegal investigations and its admissibility in court is based on experiments and scientific tests where it can be demonstrated that it is reliable and will aid in understanding the facts in dispute. In general, the requirements for admissibility of scientific evidence includes: (i) Experiments conducted under substantially similar conditions, and (ii) Expert testimony as to the reliability of the testing procedures in which the procedure was conducted by qualified experts in the field who can appear in court to testify as to the conduct of the test and the reliability of the testing procedures.
- Identification issues presented to the court often involve probabilities in which it is attempted to show that the applied technologies were properly done and were specific, sensitive, and precise, and either exclude the individual or identify the individual with reasonable certainty. These rules basically provide that unless there is some special circumstance "all relevant evidence is admissible". Proposed four "pertinent considerations" for federal trail judges to take into account whether scientific evidence is reliable: (i) Is the hypothesis set forward by the scientific expert falsifiable or testable? (ii) Has the theory or technique been subjected to peer review and publication? (ii) What is the potential rate of error in the method used? And (iv) Has the method or theory gained general acceptance, which "can be an important fact in ruling particular evidence admissible? These four questions reflect the general expectations of "scientific evidence".

CHAPTER 12 Dentist Role in Child Abuse

- Child abuse may be defined as any act of commission or omission that endangers or impairs a child's physical or emotional health and development. Such acts include physical, sexual, or emotional abuse, as well as physical neglect, inadequate supervision, and emotional deprivation. Child abuse is second only to SIDS (Sudden Infant Death Syndrome) as the leading cause of death in children under one year of age. In older children it is second only to accidents. It is now widely agreed that an absolutely crucial factor in the fight against child abuse is early recognition of the problem so that effective intervention can be undertaken.

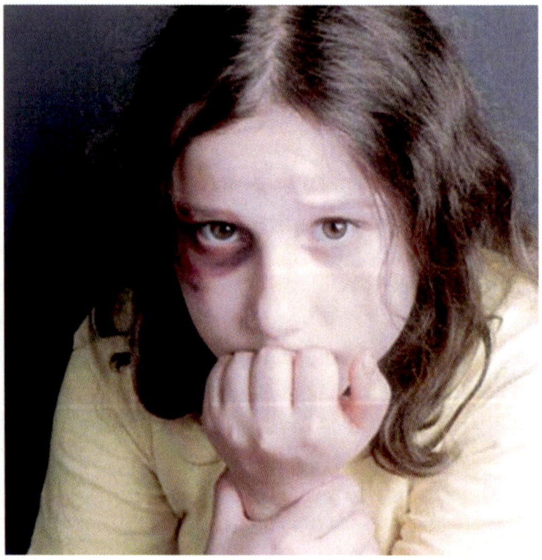

Fig. 12.1

- It is important to realize that all members of the dental team have unique opportunity—and a legal obligation—to assist in the struggle against child abuse. This special opportunity exists because a high proportion of abused children suffer injuries to the face and head, including the oral and perioral regions. These injuries may be observed during the course of dental treatment—and in some cases even before the child is seated in the dental chair. To helping dental health care workers and others fulfill an important mission – the detection and reporting of child abuse. It will also touch on the use of dental evidence in crimes against children. The ultimate goal is to save children's lives.
- Our mission involves: (i) Knowing the signs of child abuse and neglect and (ii) Fulfilling the legal and moral obligation to prevent further abuse by documenting the injuries by photographs or other means and reporting the matter to the police or social welfare agency. Whether called by the prosecution or the defense, the expert's goal should always be the same—to assist the trier of fact (the judge or the jury) in the effort to seek the truth.

INCIDENCE OF OROFACIAL LESIONS

Detecting Child Abuse in the Dental Office

- When a child presents for examination, particularly if there is an injury involved, the history may alert the dental team to the possibility of child abuse. Indeed, the history may be the single most important source of information. Because legal proceedings could follow, the history should be recorded in detail.

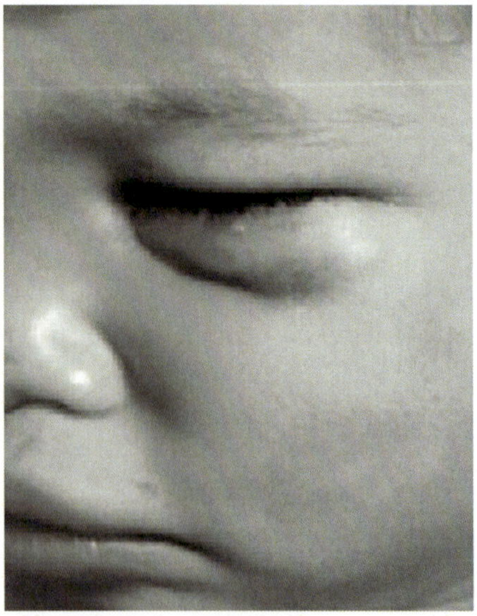

Fig. 12.2

- While one should always realize that there are other possible explanations, the possibility of child abuse or neglect should be considered whenever the history reveals the following:
  - The present injury is one of a series of injuries that the child has experienced.
  - The family offers an explanation that is not compatible with the nature of the injury.

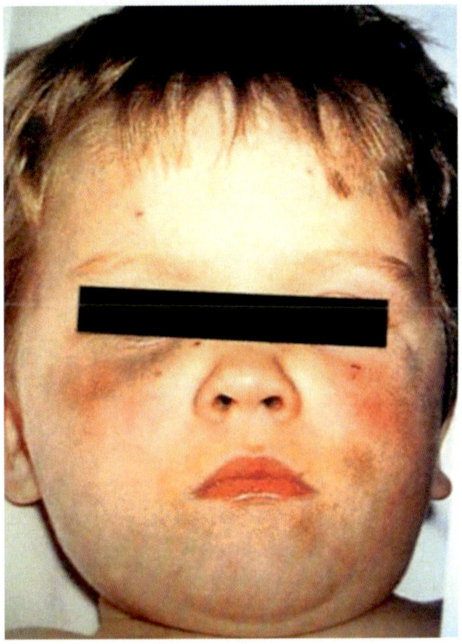

Fig. 12.3

  - There has been an extraordinary delay in seeking care for the injury.
  - The family does not want to discuss the circumstances of the injury.

While the above finding are by no means conclusive, they should cause the examiner to look further for possible signs of abuse and to consider this among the possibilities to be confirmed or eliminated.

GENERAL PHYSICAL FINDINGS

Before examining the mouth, alert members of the dental team may note general physical findings that are consistent with child abuse or neglect:

- The child's nutritional state is poor and growth is subnormal.
- Extraoral injuries are noted. They may be in various stages of healing, indicating the possibility of repeated trauma.
- Bruises may change from reddish-blue or purple to green, yellow, then brown over a period of 10 to 14+ days.
- There may be bruises or abrasions that reflect the shape of the offending object, e.g. belt buckle, strap hand.

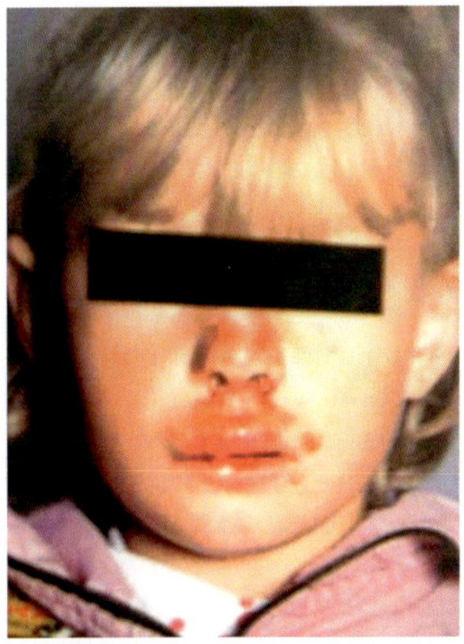

Fig. 12.4

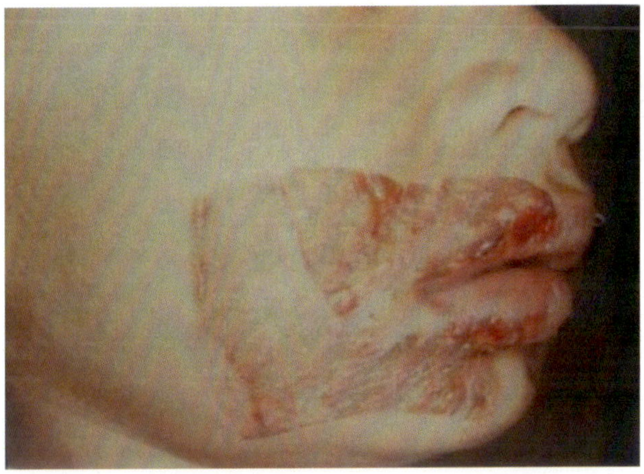

Fig. 12.5

- Cigarette burns or friction burns may be noted, e.g. from ligatures of wrists, gag on mouth.
- There may be bitemarks, bald patches (where hair has been pulled out), injuries on extremities or on the face, eyes, ears or around the mouth.

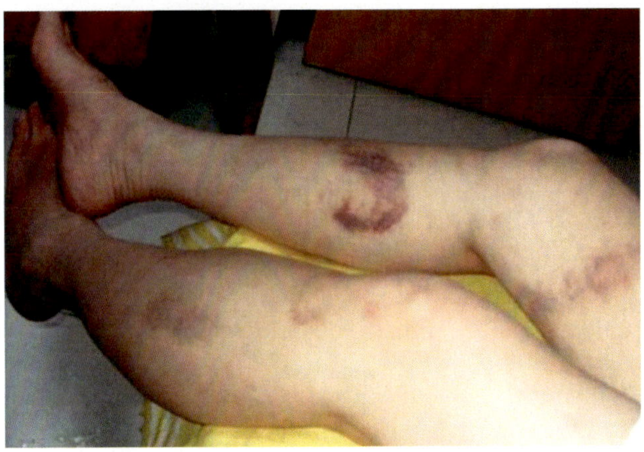

Fig. 12.6

Findings on Dental Examination

Examination of dental injuries includes thorough visual observation, radiographic studies, manipulation of the jaws, pulp vitality tests, and percussion. Transillumination may also be helpful.

TYPICAL ORAL LESIONS

Both oral and facial injuries of child abuse may occur alone or conjunction with injuries to other parts of the body. The oral lesions associated with child abuse are usually bruises, lacerations, abrasions, or fractures. Suspicion of child abuse should be particularly strong when new injuries are present along with older injuries. Thus scars, particularly on the lips, are evidence of previous trauma and should alert the investigator to the possibility of child abuse. As noted earlier, further investigation is required when the explanation for the injuries does not justify the clinical findings.

Tears of the Labial or Lingual Frenula

- Tears of the frenula, particularly the labial frenum, are frequently seen in child abuse cases. These injuries may result from blunt force trauma. For example, the labial frenum may be torn when a hand or other blunt object is forcibly applied to the upper lip to silence the child. Injuries of this type may also occur in forced feeding, as a result of the bottle being forced into the mouth.

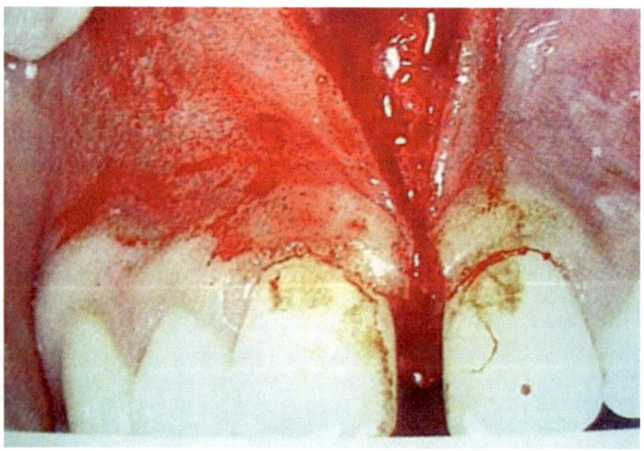

Fig. 12.7

Oral Mucosa Torn from Gingiva

- Blunt force trauma to the lower face may also cause the mucosal lining of the inner surface of the lip to be torn away from the gingival. A forceful slap, for example, may have this effect. The location and extent of the injury will depend on the magnitude of force and the location and direction of the blow.
- Severe trauma to the lower face may loosen teeth, completely displace them from their alveolar sockets, and/or cause dental fractures. It is not uncommon for root fractures to occur, but this finding may be missed unless the radiographs are examined carefully.
- These injuries, as well as most other traumatic injuries, may be accidental rather than abusive. Therefore, one must always determine whether the injury is compatible with the explanation given. If the dental injuries resulted from a fall, for example, one would usually expect to also find bruised or abraded knees, hands, or elbows. When these additional injuries are not present, further inquiry is appropriate.

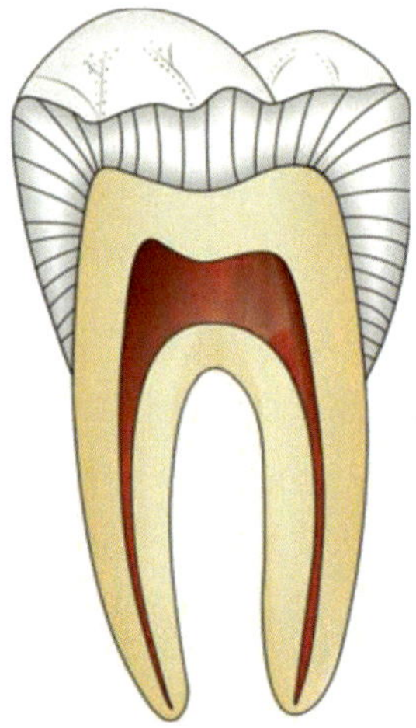

Fig. 12.8

- In evaluating and reporting dental injuries. It may be helpful to use Andersen's classification, based on a system adopted by the World Health Organization. It is summarized below:
  - Crown infarction—incomplete (crack) of enamel with loss of tooth substance.

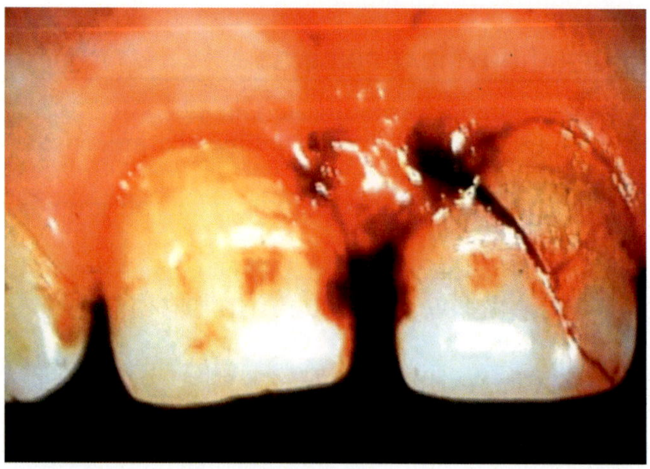

Fig. 12.9

- Uncomplicated crown fracture—confined to enamel or enamel and dentin, pulp not exposed.
- Complicated crown fracture—involves enamel and dentin, pulp is exposed
- Uncomplicated crown—root fracture—involves enamel, dentin, and cementum, but does not expose pulp

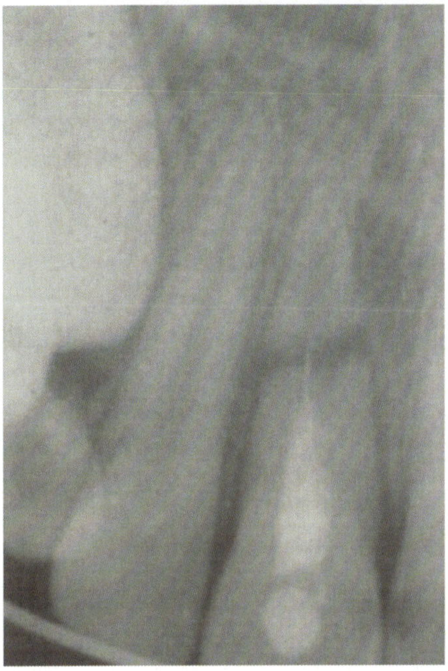

Fig. 12.10

- Complicated crown-root fracture-involves enamel, dentin, cementum, and exposes pulp
- Concussion—injury to supporting structures without abnormal loosening or displacement of the tooth, but with marked reaction to percussion.
- Subluxation (loosening)—injury to supporting structures with abnormal loosening, but without displacement of the tooth
- Intrusive luxation—tooth displaced into alveolar bone, injury accompanied by comminution or fracture of alveolar socket
- Extrusive luxation—tooth partially displaced out of its socket
- Lateral luxation—tooth displaced in a direction other than axially, with comminution or fracture of alveolar socket
- Exarticulation (complete avulsion)—tooth completely avulsed from socket
- Comminution of alveolar socket—Crushing and compression of alveolar socket, found with intrusive and lateral luxation.

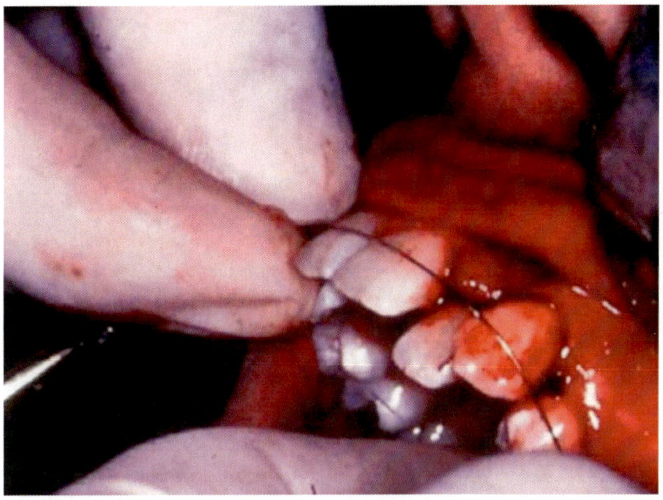

Fig. 12.11

- Fracture of mandible or maxilla—involves the base of mandible or maxilla and often the alveolar process, may or may not involve alveolar socket
- Laceration of gingival or oral mucosa—shallow or deep wound in mucosa resulting from tear, and normally produced by sharp object
- Contusion of gingiva or oral mucosa—superficial wound produced by rubbing or scraping mucosa, leaving raw, bleeding surface.

Darkened and/or Nonvital Teeth

- The tissues of the dental pulp receive their primary blood supply through the apical foramen. When the tooth receives a concussion, the apical blood vessels may be severed, or hematoma or edema may occlude the blood vessels as they enter the tooth. As a consequence, the pulp may become necrotic and nonvital. Necrosis of the previously pink pulp tissues will usually cause a noticeable darkening of the tooth.
- In some cases of dental trauma, the dental pulp's response to the injury may be to deposit additional secondary dentin in the pulp chamber. This may continue until the entire pulp chamber is filled in, or obtunded. Again, the loss of the hollow pulp chamber with its normally pinkish contents is likely to cause a change in the color of the tooth.
- It is important to remember that both of the processes described above occur over a period of weeks, or even months. Consequently, when a child presents with current dental trauma and also has one or more dark teeth unrelated to caries, it is probable that the child has experienced previous trauma. Further inquiry to determine the nature of the trauma should be undertaken.

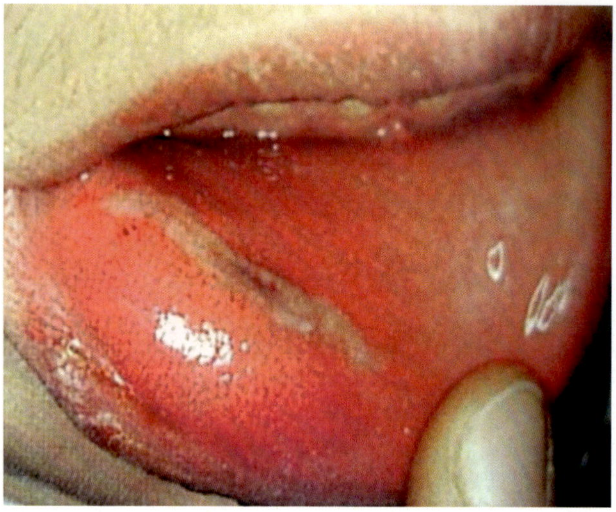

Fig. 12.12

Previously Missing Teeth

In examining a child who has experienced recent trauma, it may be noted that one or more teeth has been lost prior to the present incident. The etiology of this earlier tooth loss should be investigated. If it was due to "an accident", a pattern of repeated trauma has been established. This pattern needs to be evaluated, and child abuse is one of the possibilities to be considered.

Trauma to the Lip

It is not uncommon to find contusions, lacerations, burns, or scars on the lips of abused children. Bruises to the lip may result from forced feeding. Burns on the lip, as well as burns on the face of tongue, may be signs of physical punishment. Bruises at the angles of the mouth may result from efforts to gag or silence a child.

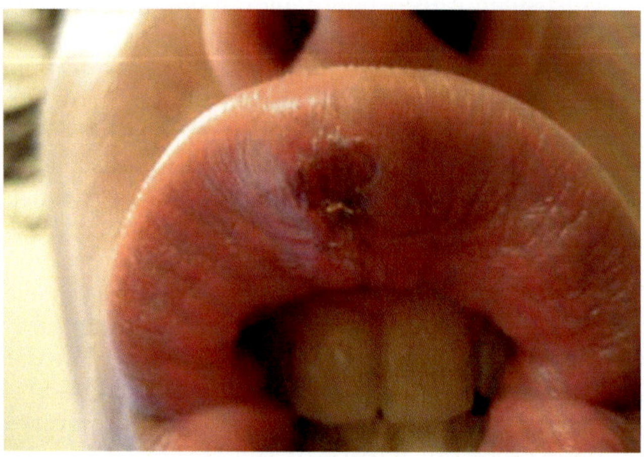

Fig. 12.13

Trauma to the Tongue

The tongue of an abused child may exhibit abnormal anatomy or function due to scarring. This may result from a burn or other trauma.

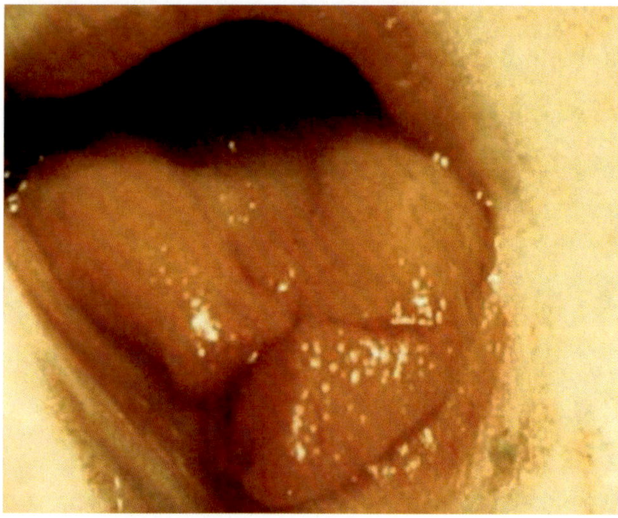

Fig. 12.14

Other Soft Tissue Injuries

Trauma to the mouth may also cause ulceration of the palate or uvula. Additionally, lacerations are sometimes found in the floor of the mouth, which may be caused by forced bottle feeding.

FRACTURES OF JAWS AND ASSOCIATED STRUCTURES

- Fractures of the maxilla, mandible, and other cranial bones may be found in cases of child abuse. If the radiologic study shows signs of old as well as new fractures, a pattern of repeated trauma has been found, and needs to be investigated with reference to possible child abuse.
- The examination for maxillofacial fractures is performed within the concept of overall patient care, including airway maintenance, control of hemorrhage, and neurologic examination. In a significant number of jaw fractures there is also damage to associated structures, including the cribriform plate, nasal, and zygomatic bones. Intracranial lesions and skull fractures may also be present.
- The diagnosis of fractures of the jaws is made primarily on the basis of clinical and radiographic findings. The clinical examination includes both extraoral and intraoral palpation. Bilateral palpation is helpful to detect asymmetry.

- Swelling or ecchymosis in the lower face is suggestive of fractures of the mandible. Fractures should also be suspected if there is an abrupt change in the occlusal level of the teeth. This may be associated with open bite, difficulty in opening the mouth, and facial asymmetry. Other signs and symptoms include abnormal mobility of bony structures, or the ability to move the mandible beyond its normal excursion in any direction. Supporting the angle of the mandible and pressing the anterior mandibular region up and down to detect fractures of the body of the mandible. Crepitation and deviation of the midline on closing may be diagnostic signs, as well. Pain in the area of the temporomandibular joints may suggest fractures in this region.

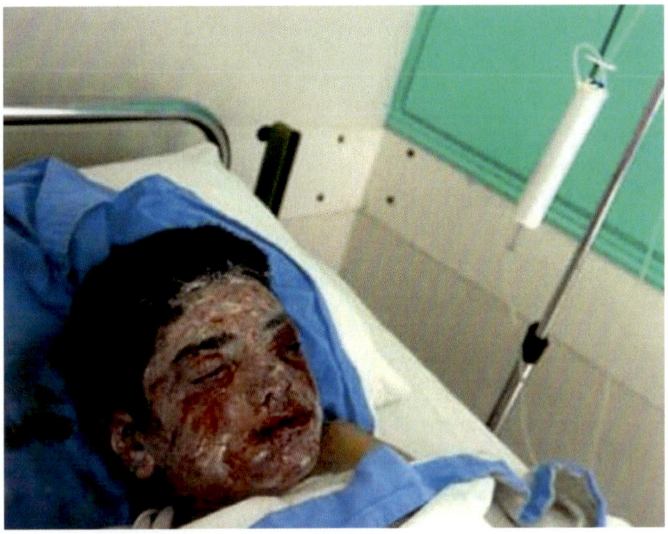

Fig. 12.15

- The medical practitioner who observes dental trauma is well advised to seek consultation with a dentist experienced in dental injuries to children. This might be a pediatric dentist, oral and maxillofacial surgeon, or general dentist. This added expertise is important, not only to care for the present injury, but also to help evaluate previous trauma.

GENERAL NEGLECT OF THE MOUTH

A child with rampant, untreated dental decay and poor oral hygiene is suffering from significant neglect. The consequences may be pain, infection, and a threat to the child's general health and well-being. The medical or dental practitioner who observes this condition, particularly if it continues after having been brought to the attention of the parents, should realize that the situation is no different than having parents neglect in any other important medical condition. Moreover, this

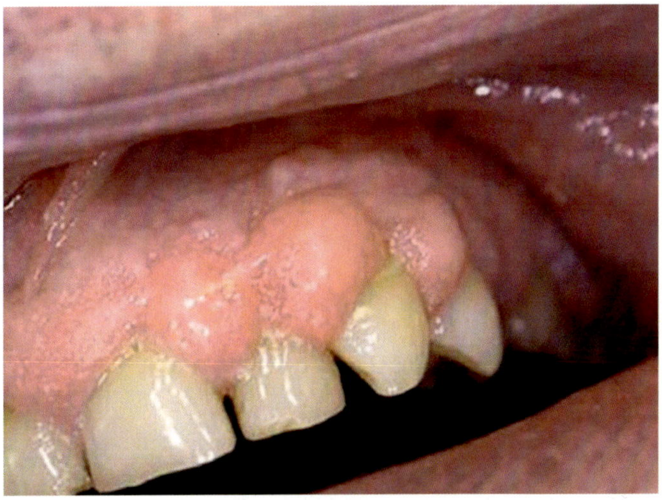

Fig. 12.16

may be a sign of a more generalized problem in caring for the child. Indeed, Blain reports that a preliminary study supports the high correlation between dental neglect and CAN (child abuse and neglect).

The following conditions should be considered reasons for reporting if the caretaker consciously fails to follow treatment recommendations in potentially life-threatening situations:

- Failure to provide prescribed antibiotics.
- Failure to seek treatment for cellulites and its associated infections.
- Failure to seek treatment for any acute or chronic infection, including dental caries, when underlying life-threatening system conditions are present such as subacute bacterial endocarditis, glomerulonephritis, or juvenile-onset diabetes.
- In addition, consideration should be given to reporting the following conditions if the dental situation is deteriorating to the point where irreversible harm will be done, leading to pain, discomfort, or a decrease in health or welfare.
- Diagnosed caries or periodontal diseases which have been referred for treatment and caretakers have failed to keep appointments.
- Presence of untreated traumatic injuries as indicated by nonvital teeth, avulsed permanent teeth, and injuries to soft tissues, including signs of scarring.
- Failure to seek recommended treatment for diagnosed severe malrelationships of the maxilla and mandible, including craniofacial anomalies, which may result in deficient speech, esthetic deformities, and psychological disturbances.
- In cases of suspected child abuse, in descending order of frequency, were fractures of the teeth (32%), oral

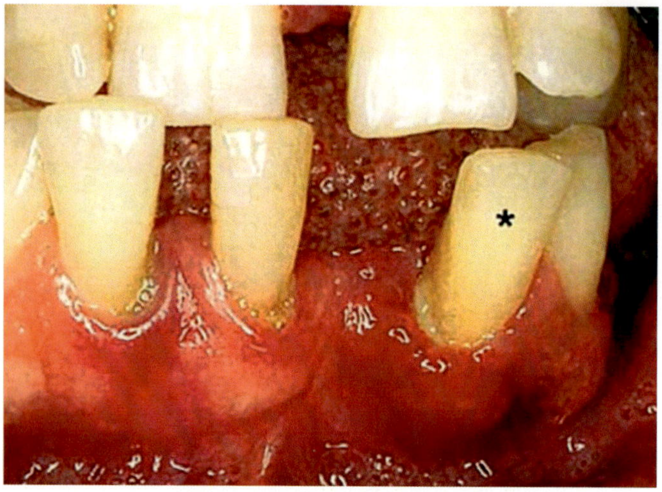

Fig. 12..17

bruises (24%), oral lacerations (14%), fractures of the mandible or maxilla (11%), and oral burns (5%). However, other authors report that lesions in which the oral mucosa is torn away from the gingival may be the most common injury to the face, and may occur in as many as 50% of child abuse cases.

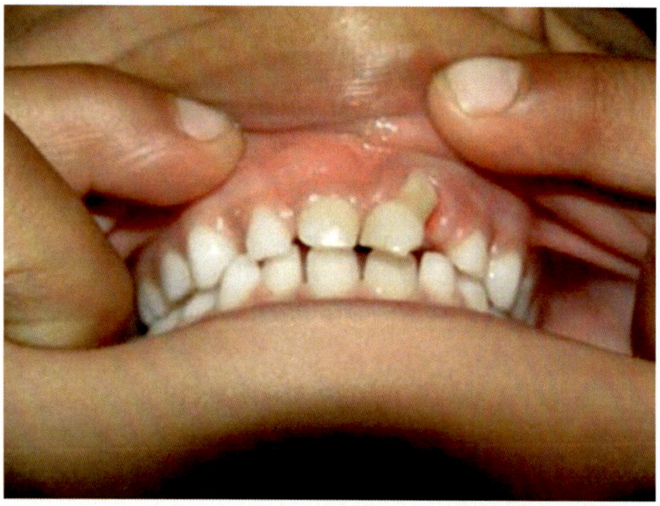

Fig. 12.18

- Becker et al reported that of the 14 cases in their series with intraoral injuries, 43% were contusions and ecchymoses, 28.5% were abrasions and lacerations, and 28.5% were dental trauma.

ASSOCIATED FACIAL LESIONS

- Becker et al found that in their series of facial injuries in abused children, 66% of the injuries werecontusions and ecchymoses, 28% were abrasions and lacerations, 3% were burns, 2% were fractures, and 1% were bites.

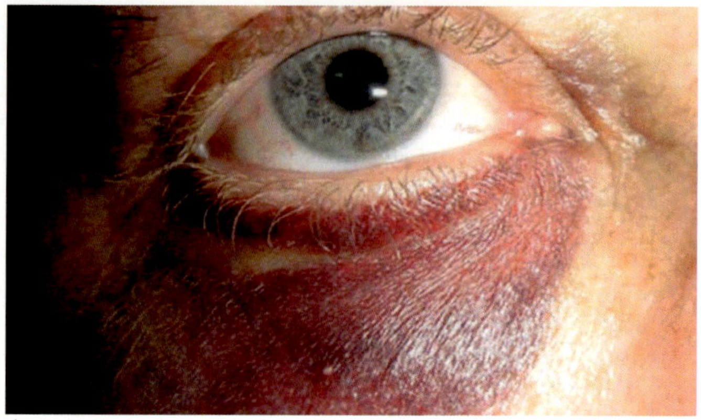

Fig. 12.19

- Knowledge of the color changes associated with bruising may be important in determining when the injury occurred, and in determining whether other injuries occurred during the same event or at different times. Kessler and Hyden point out that after the injury occurs, the area is usually tender and swollen, but the bruise may not be visible as a contusion or ecchymosis for 24 to 72 hours. A reddish-blue or purple color may change to green in 5 to 7 days, then to yellow in 7 to 10 days, then to brown in 10 to 14 + days, before clearing 2 to 4 weeks.
- Injuries to the face may include trauma to the eyes, ears, and nose, as well as to the oral cavity. Blunt force trauma to the eye may cause periorbital bruises (black eyes), acute hyphema (blood in the anterior chamber of the eye), retinal and subconjunctival hemorrhage,

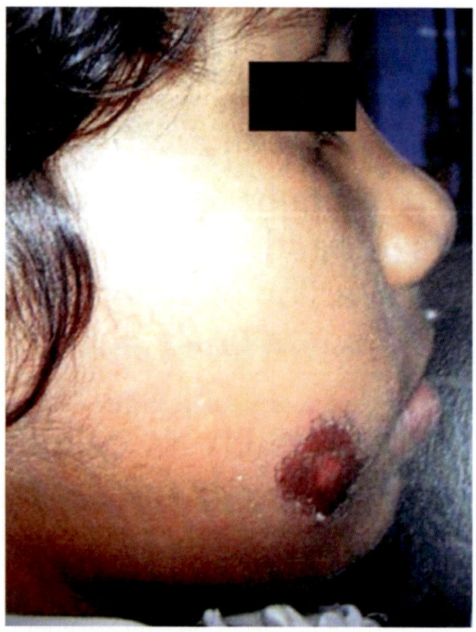

Fig. 12.20

ruptured globe, dislocated lens, optic atrophy, traumatic cataract, and detached retina.

- Direct trauma to the nose may cause deviated septum due to cartilage injury or hematoma formation. Such trauma may also cause nasal fractures, with accompanying bilateral ecchymosis. Injuries to the ear may be associated with twisting and bruising, while repeated blows may eventually result in a "cauliflower ear". Blows to the ear can also rupture the tympanic membrane or cause hemorrhage and hematoma formation.
- Bruises from hand slapping are not uncommon. In such cases the bruise may reproduce the outline of the hand in startling detail. As noted earlier, other cutaneous injuries may also take the shape of the object used to inflict the injury, such as a belt buckle or looped electric cord.
- It has been suggested that whenever bruises occur on both sides of the mouth or face at once, or if there is scarring of the lips, abuse should be suspected. Also, the presence of injuries on multiple body surfaces suggests abuse. McNeese and Hebeler point out that such multiplanar injuries would occur accidentally only as a result of tumbling falls (e.g. falling down stairs) or trauma incurred during automobile accidents.
- As noted earlier, the lips and corners of the mouth may show contusions, lacerations, burns, or scars due to the frequency of attack to the mouth in abused children. In the author's experience, bitemarks on the face of children are most commonly found on or around the cheeks. However, they may occur on the ear, nose, chin, or elsewhere.

DOCUMENTING AND REPORTING CHILD ABUSE

- When one suspects child abuse, it is important to document the findings thoroughly. This record of the evidence is crucial for whatever legal proceeding may follow. Documentation may involve written notes, photographs, and radiographs. In some cases videotapes or audiotapes may be helpful. It is important that critical photographs of injuries include a ruler or scale held adjacent to the injury and on the same plane as the injured surface. When possible, 35-mm photography should be used. Fortunately, cameras equipped for dental photography are ideal for photographing most body injuries.
- It the child requires medical attention, referral should be made to the proper resource. Even if immediate medical care is not required, if a pediatrician is readily available the dentist may wish to consult regarding the suspected child abuse prior to reporting. However, the absence of consultation does not relieve the dentist from the responsibility to promptly report suspected abuse.

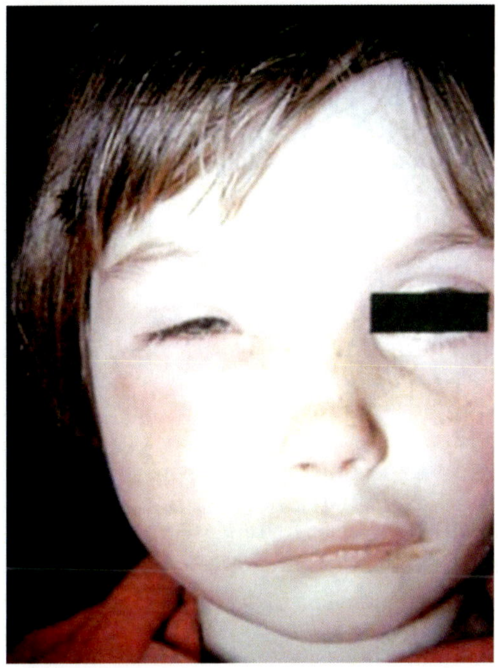

Fig. 12.21

- In the great majority of states, dentists, as health professionals, are required by law to report suspected cases of child abuse and neglect, and a penalty is provided for failure to report.
- To illustrate the reporting requirement, California law requires that any child-care custodian, health practitioner, nonmedical practitioner, or employee of a child protective agency who has knowledge of, or who observes a child whom he or she suspects has been the victim of child abuse, report to a child protective agency immediately or as soon as possible and send a written report within 36 hours of learning of the incident. The definition of Health Practitioner includes dentist resident, dental hygienist, and other licensed individuals, which includes the registered dental assistant.
- The report can be made to the local police agency or welfare department. To a local agency or for other supportive information.
- In addition to criminal liability for failure to report, the practitioner could also face a civil lawsuit, if there is subsequent injury to the child.
- In general, most states provide broad legal protection for health care practitioners who report child abuse. While lawsuits can still be brought against the reporter, they are likely to be dismissed under the immunity statutes.

PROBLEMS IN DENTAL REPORTING OF CHILD ABUSE

- It is generally agreed that the true number of child abuse cases is probably far in excess of the number of cases actually reported. Since a substantial number of abused children have injuries in or around the mouth, it would seek likely that dentists would be a significant source of child abuse reporting.
- The most common reason given for unwillingness to report was uncertainty about the diagnosis, fear of litigation, unfamiliarity with symptoms of child abuse, possible effect on the practice, reluctance to believe one could inflict cruelties on one's off spring, and uncertainty, about the reliability of the child's account of the injury. Significantly, the overwhelming majority felt they had inadequate timing in the diagnosis of child abuse, and many who were surveyed stated that they would be interested in obtaining additional information of the project. Dental professionals may be negligent in their and social roles of preventing and intervening in cases of CAN. "This failure to report cases of child abuse violates state reporting laws; not reporting cases may, in effect, allow the continuation of child abuse, and more importantly, prevent both the child and his family from getting the social welfare and medical aid that they may need. Low rate of reporting among dentists is smilar to the low rate of physicians reporting confirmed abuse cases.
- It should be noted that in recent years efforts have been made to educate the dental profession and encourage appropriate reporting.

OVERDIAGNOSIS OF CHILD ABUSE

- The importance of reporting suspected cases of child abuse and neglect cannot be overemphasized, the thoughtful practitioner should also consider the other side of the coin. When a child's problem is thought to be child abuse and it is not, considerable harm may be done to the child, the parents and the doctor-patient relationship. They included a child whose generalized bruises were later found to be related to cystic fibrosis. Overdiagnosing the battered child syndrome can be as harmful as failing to consider it.
- In an interesting recent case, physicians noted vaginal discharge in a nine-year-old girl. They suspected sexual abuse. The child was taken from the parents that same day and placed in protective custody for seven weeks. It was later determined that the discharge was due to chickenpox, rather that child abuse. The parents then sued the physician, hospital, and others.
- It is important for the dental team to be familiar will certain cultural practices that may produce lesions similar to those of child abuse. For example, children from Vietnamese families may present with ecchymotic lesions involving not only the back, but the face as well. These lesions may be produced by pinching the skin, or by rubbing it with a coarse cloth. This is part of the practice intended to free the body of "bad winds", believed responsible for various illnesses. The practice has been described as "pseudobattering" because the intent is to help rather than harm the child.

CHAPTER

13 Teaching Forensic Odontology

INTRODUCTION

- Sustained Education and demand over the past half-century has rendered forensic odontology a valuable component of forensic investigatons in many countries. Forensic odontologists are routinely consulted for assistance in legal and criminal problems. Moreover, forensic odontology has made great strides in the last decade, ranging from two-to three-dimensional digital analysis of bitemarks to extracting DNA from teeth for the purpose of identification. This is a reflection of dentists' willingness to contribute to the community in ways other than preventive and therapeutic service. However, in the wake of recent advances, it may be useful to re-examine the purpose, constituents and approach of education in the forensic odontology.

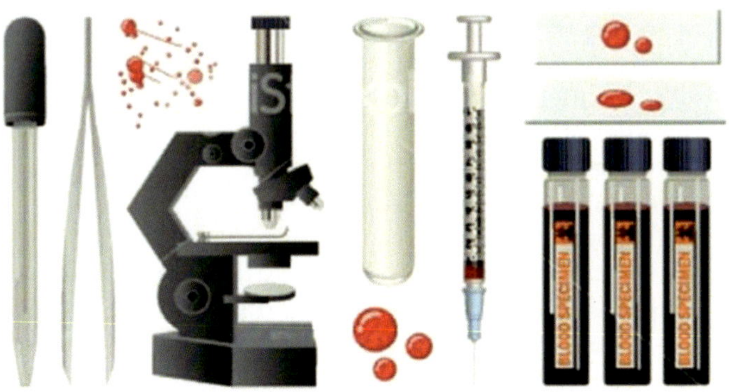

Fig. 13.1

HISTORY OF TEACHING FORENSIC ODONTOLOGY

- The application of dental sciences in criminal and legal investigations gathered momentum in the West during the 1950s and 1960s. The associated need for formal training in forensic odontology and its inclusion in dental curricula, was recognized and acted on in the 1960s and 1970s. The discipline had been practiced by individuals much earlier than this and the first course in forensic dentistry was probably conducted by Prof Sadanori Mita of Japan as early as 1903. The correspondence course outlined 'methods of examination, evaluation and classification of bitemarks and the differences between ante- and post-mortem appearances'. This course subsequently formed the basis of his lectures at Tokyo Dental College between 1922 and 1936.
- Undergraduate forensic odontology education in North America dates back to the early 1960s, while in the UK, it has been taught since the early 1970s. The first postgraduate program in forensic odontology in the USA was conducted by the Armed Forces Institute of Pathology in 1963, while in continental Europe, a postgraduate course was first offered in Copenhagen in May 1979.

THE NEED TO TEACH FORENSIC ODONTOLOGY

- The legendary Gosta Gustafson stated that it is essential... that a course in forensic odontology should form part of the basic undergraduate curriculum'. Salley felt that knowledge of forensic odontology among dentists is essential to better understand the intricacies and subtleties specific to forensic science and criminal investigation. Dentists may be consulted on occasion for assistance in postmortem dental identification, disaster victim identification, age estimation and criminal cases involving bitemark evidence. Hence, the dental graduate should have a wide-ranging knowledge of theoretical and practical aspects of forensic odontology.
- Be reasonably competent to recognize forensic cases with dental applications when consulted by the police, forensic pathologists, lawyers and associated professionals
- Be capable of proper collection of dental evidence related to cases of identification, ethnic and sex differentiation, age-estimation and bitemarks

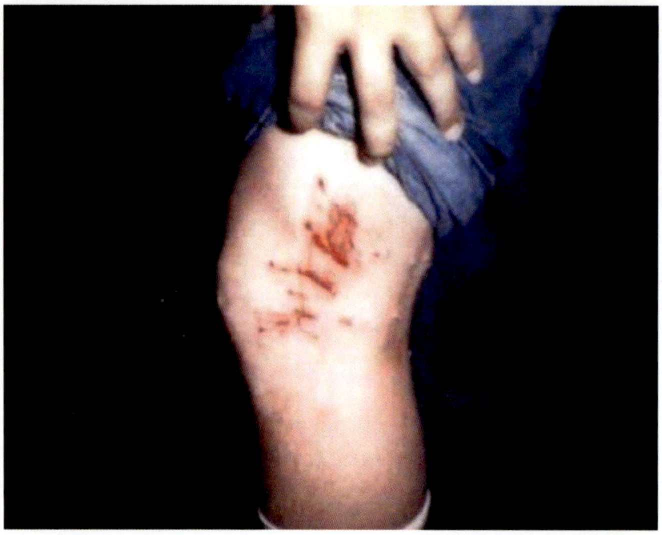

Fig. 13.2

- Be able to assist qualified forensic odontologists in analysis, evaluation and presentation of dental facts within the realm of law
- Teaching forensic odontology to undergraduates should ensure that dentists are able to assist forensic investigations if, and when the need arises.

What are the constituents of forensic odontology?

- What constitutes the curricular needs for teaching forensic odontoloygy. Topics such as: (i) Postmortem dental identification and disaster victim identification, (ii) Age-estimation, (iii) Anthropology, and (iv) Bitemark analysis, are covered in all the universities.

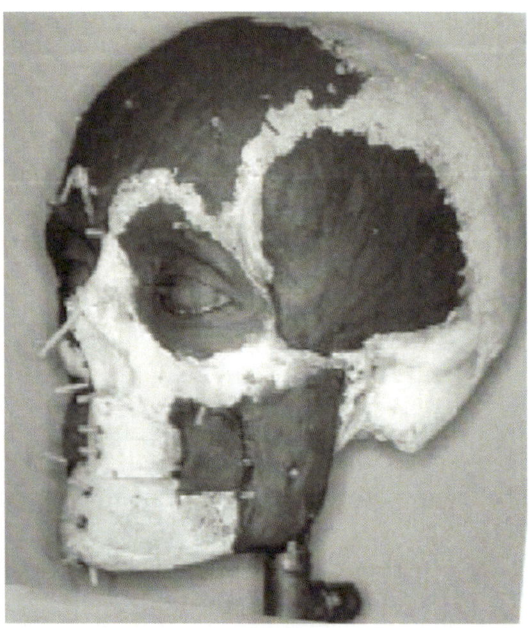

Fig. 13.3

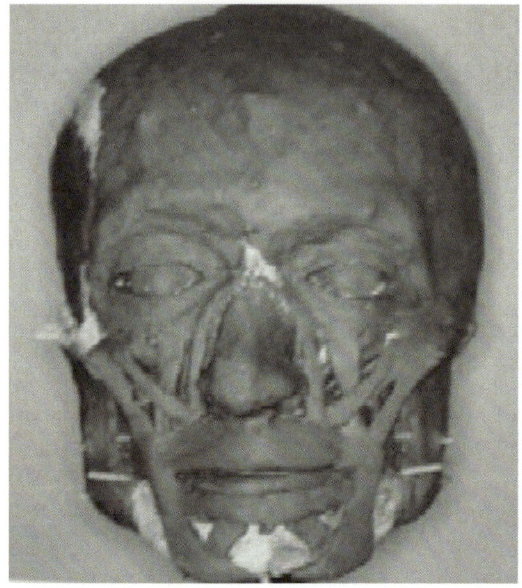

Fig. 13.4

- Postmortem dental identification, which includes identification of decomposed, traumatized or burned remains, is regarded as the most important aspect of forensic odontology. In fact, the genesis of modern forensic odontology could be attributed to the use of dental evidence in identifying victims of two European disasters of the 19th century: The fire at the Ring Theatre of Vienna in 1881 which claimed 449 lives, and the Bazaar de la Charite fire of Paris in 1897 that resulted in 127 casualties.
- The dentition has long been used for estimating age. In the first half of 19th century the Factory Act of England prevented a child without the second permanent molar from working in factories. The tables of Schour and Massler and Gustafson's method, two early scientific estimators of age that utilized teeth, date back >50 years.
- Anthropological examination of teeth can yield information useful in building the profile of unidentified individuals, e.g. Lund and Mornstad suggested that tooth measurements could indicate sex, while morphological features such as Carabelli's trait give clues to a person's ethnicity.
- Bitemark investigation is probably the most challenging aspect of forensic odontology. Its judicious use can prove critical in sexual assault, homicide and other criminal investigations.
- Interpretation of antemortem dental records is a crucial part of dental identification. The ability to decipher terminologies, short-hands and notations used by dentists from different parts of the world is essential to successfully match the dental record to the postmortem data.

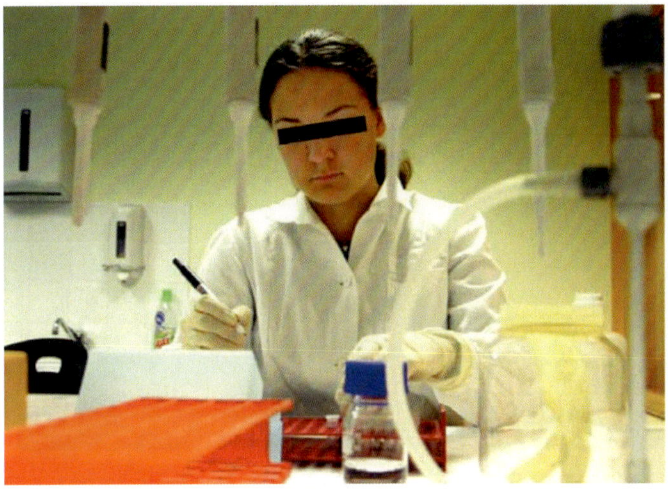

Fig. 13.5

- To the general practitioner not used to the practical details of court procedures, the possibility of testifying in court can be intimidating. Therefore, session(s) on the dentists' role as a expert witness and mock court trials can be an invaluable prelude to real-life situations.
- While the value of skull-face superimposition in identification is debatable, it is a useful adjunct in identifying skeletal specimens in the absence of antemortem dental records.
- Topics such as dental record interpretation, the dentists' role as an expert witness, and extraoral identification methods such as skull-face superimposition are covered at the majority of the institutes.
- In addition to these topics, specific aspects of forensic odontology are emphasized in individual institutions. In the University of Oslo, Norway, as many as five lectures and two 3 hr seminars are devoted to dental jurisprudence and ethics. In one of the seminars, students are given cases where problems have occurred or could occur, and they discuss what they would do under such situations in their own practice. Recognising the need for forensic odontologists to prepare injury reports, a lecture on dental injuries and a court case involving the same is organized.
- Of particular interest are the lectures on animal dentition and lip prints. A lecture 'structure of the court system' is taken by a lawyer attached to the attorney-general's office. In fact, some argue that special lectures which include professionals from other aspects of forensic analysis and dental identification, respectively, and it is felt imperative that students are exposed to the basics of such procedures. Third year dental undergraduates are taught forensic odontology and forensic medicine. Forensic medicine makes up a major component and, in addition to lectures (termed 'structured interactive session' or SIS), include practical exercises in soft tissue examination, examination of weapons, toxicology, injury report writing and autopsies. The philosophy behind teaching detailed forensic medicine to dental undergraduates is that dentsist should be able to assist routine medicolegal cases, particularly since some of this country's regions are geographically isolated, with minimal health professional available.

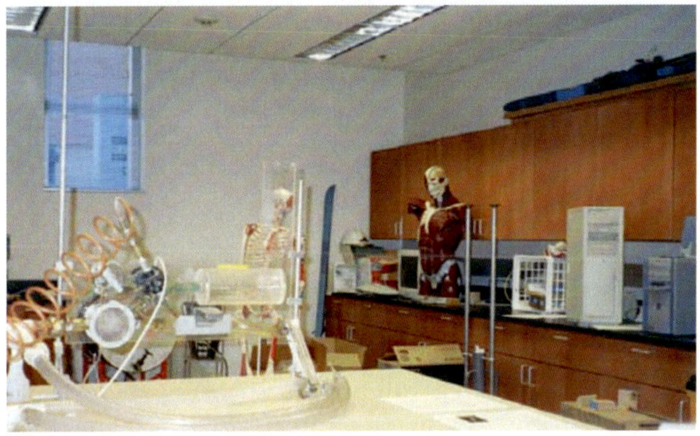

Fig. 13.6

- Practical exercises in forensic odontology include postmortem dental examination, simulated dental identification and disaster victim identification, radiographi age estimation, craniomandibular sex differences, as well as bitemark evidence collection and analysis. The latter makes use of two-dimensional digital analysis suggested by Johansen and Bowers, making the exercise more exciting for students.
- Animal dentition and lip prints are also covered. While some may be surprised at the inclusion of animal dental patterns inforensic odontology, a basic knowledge of comparative dental anatomy is essential in investigating cases of animal bitemarks. This has great relevance in frequent cases of carnivorous attacks on the fringes of nature may necessitate accurate identification of the species or individual animal. The investigation of latent lip prints is analogous to fingerprint analysis, and can be considered a genuine subspecialty of forensic odontology; however, a lack of routine casework and research seems to preclude its detailed coverage.
- While relevant aspects of forensic odontology are integral to the institutes surveyed, insufficient coverage of DNA techniques in most of these institutes may deprive students of exposure to frontier forensic science. That stated it does not imply the non-existence of institutes that teach these topics. The author

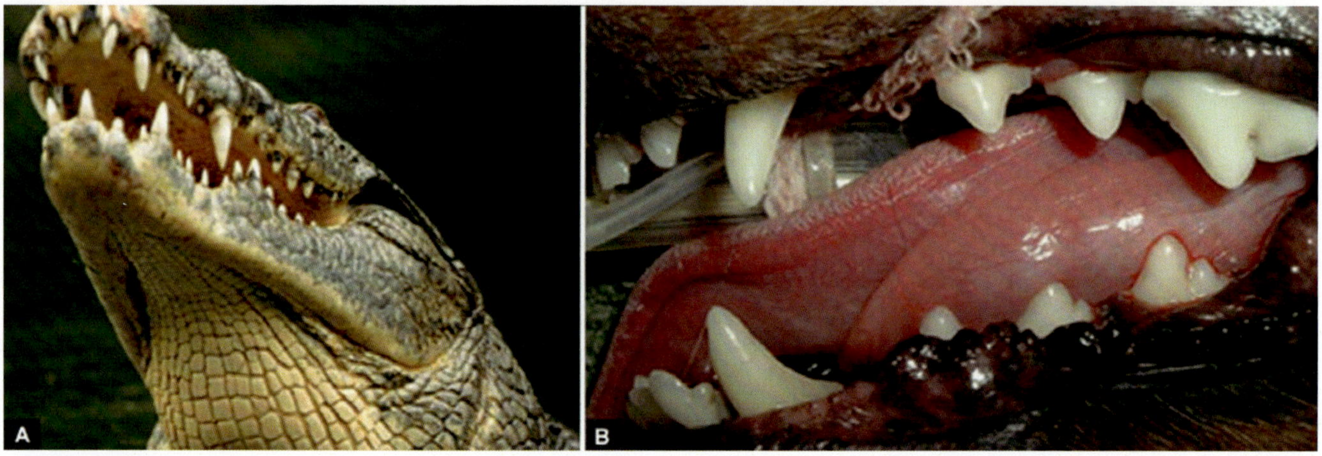

Figs 13.7A and B

recognizes that the institutes surveyed do not necessarily represent their respective countries, and at least two of the specialists surveyed have indicated that the programs are specific to their universities. St suggest the dentists to (i) Recognize forensic cases with dental implications; and (ii) Assist forensic odontologists in routine casework. Scientific knowledge and medical knowledge advance as the years go on... Forensic odontology has evolved and its importance in police investigation is widely acknowledged by the general public and legal authorities. It is essential that the curriculum content is constantly updated for the benefit of the discipline and the community it serves. This ensures that undergraduates are aware of new trends in the subject and also enables more objective decision–making by prospective post-graduates. It is stressed that the preceding forensic odontology curricula do not represent the global norm. Hence, an in depth analysis of trends in teaching forensic odontology is possible only after undertaking a more comprehensive worldwide survey.

CHAPTER 14 Narcoanalysis

- Narcoanalysis is steadily being mainstreamed into investigations, court hearings, and laboratories in India. However, it raises serious scientific, legal, and ethical questions. These need to be addressed urgently before the practice spreads further.
- Narcoanalysis has become an increasingly, perhaps alarmingly, common term in India. It refers to the process of psychotherapy conducted on a subject by inducing a sleep-like state with the aid of barbiturates or other drugs. In a spate of high profile cases, such as those of the Nithari killers and the Mumbai train blasts, suspects have been whisked away to undergo an interview drugged with the **barbiturate sodium pentothal**.
- This practice has also garnered support from certain State governments as well as the judiciary. The Home Ministry's Directorate of Forensic Sciences plans to expand narcoanalysis facilities nationwide.
- It would appear that the narcoanalysis has acquired a life of its own. It is increasingly knocking at the doors of courts and finding ready acceptance as a device to get at the truth during police investigations, though its scientific basis and value are under strong challenge. It is for this reason that the scientific, legal, and evidentiary issues relevant to the narcoanalysis debate need to be critically discussed.
- Narcoanalysis is rarely used for therapeutic purposes today. It is surely significant that while 'truth serums' have been in use since the early part of the 20th century, they are not used in most developed countries today. During and after the War years, United States armed forces and intelligence agencies continued to experiment with truth drugs. While truth drugs can be useful in overcoming resistance not dissolved by other methods, the actual content of what comes out during the interrogation can be "psychotic manifestations ... hallucinations, illusions, delusions or disorientation.
- Studies have shown that persons who make truthful confessions are those who were likely to confess had

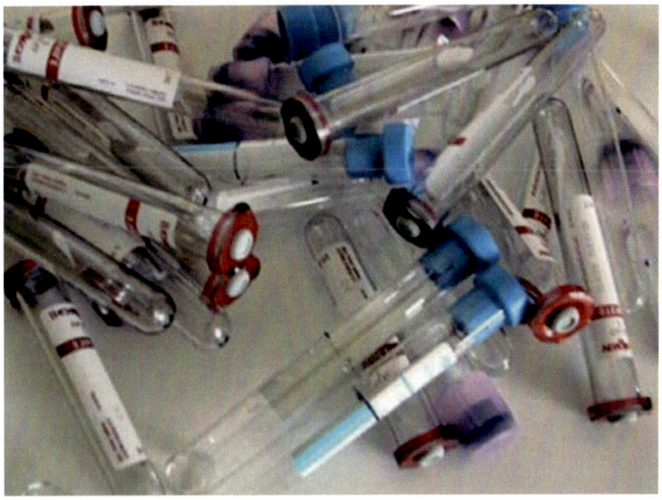

Fig. 14.1

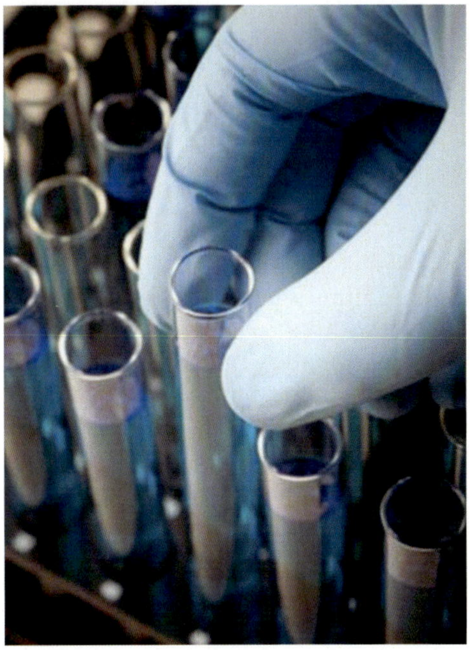

Fig. 14.2

interrogators persisted with regular methods; and that persons who lie can continue to manifest a lie even under the influence of a so called truth serum. Moreover, the investigator can induce and communicate his own thoughts and feelings to the suspect. The scientific literature indicates that if narcoanalysis has any extratherapeutic uses, it may be in making a suspect feel that he has revealed more than he actually did. With repeated questioning, it may be possible to reduce ambiguities although these cannot be eliminated.

- Scientific scepticism and the absence of controlled studies have not deterred Indian investigating agencies from running to the FSL in Gandhinagar or, more likely, Bengaluru — the narcoanalysis hub for various police departments across the country. FSL, Bengaluru, conducts sodium pentothal narcoanalysis in conjunction with three other tests — psychological profiling, polygraph ('lie-detector') tests, and brain mapping. Polygraph tests, which one can learn to 'pass' or 'fail', are used for screening and confirmation purposes only. Brain mapping, a premature if promising technique not entirely free from controversy itself, indicates whether a subject's brain stores experiential knowledge about a certain object. Narcoanalysis is used when investigators need oral elicitations from a suspect. For instance, if brain mapping indicates that the suspect stores information about a blue get away car allegedly used in the crime, the narcoanalysis, according to the FSL, Bengaluru, is used to provide information such as the number of the car, where it is parked, and so on. Narcoanalysis has a 96 to 97 % total success rate. Included in the definition of total success rate' is the discovery of information that either triggers a relevant section of the law or may be cross verified with other tests (such as brain mapping). Findings that discredit narcoanalysis are usually based on studies of scopolamine and sodium amytal and are not applicable to sodium amytal and are not applicable to sodium pentothal, which is used by the Indian laboratories. He adds that during narcoanalysis the tendency is to sleep if not questioned, rather than hallucinating or fantasizing. There are two problems with this argument. Using sodium pentothal is not a new advance in narcoanalysis. Internationally the psychological fraternity has used sodium pentothal for decades; and discontinued its use in all but the rarest cases, partly because there is no guarantee that the drug will elicit factually accurate information. It is difficult to manifest fantasies in narcoanalysis is questionable. False memory is an extremely well-researched area. While patients under narcoanalysis may find it difficult to lie consciously depending on the depth of the narcoanalysis, they can say things that are not true and on the surface of their minds. The case of a suspect who is repeatedly accused of a crime during regular interrogation, "The same thing goes on during the narcoanalysis.

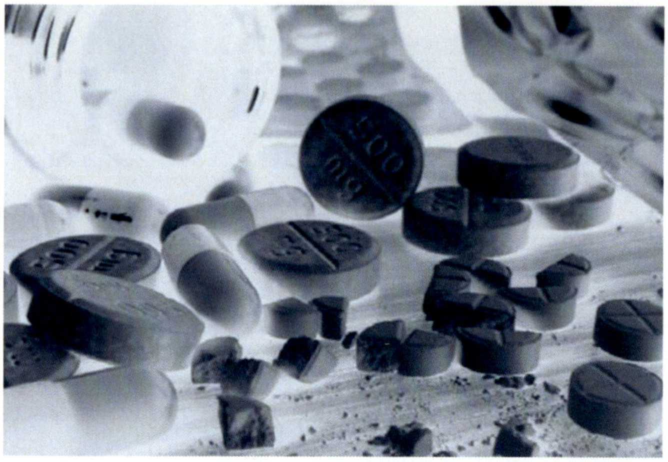

Fig. 14.3

- When science has outpaced the development of law or at least the layperson's understanding of it, there are unavoidable complexities regarding what can be admitted as evidence in court.
- We must give narcoanalysis its due and grant that it has provided valuable leads to the police in some instances. It is logically consistent for even a pseudo science to produce reliable outcomes in particular cases. The overall reliability and science behind the practice can only be determined after statistical analysis of a sufficiently large sample.
- The irony of the situation we face in India is that the science behind narcoanalysis, as we know it, has not leap-frogged the courts by any stretch of imagination. The Bengaluru research results and methods have been neither peer-reviewed nor published. The feedback that goes into defining the success of the analysis is provided in part by police questionnaires.

LEGAL ASPECTS

- Subjecting an accused to narcoanalysis is not tantamount to testimony by compulsion. The court said about the accused: "he may be taken to the laboratory for such test against his will, but the revelation during such tests is quite voluntary". There are two fallacies in this reasoning. First, if narcoanalysis is all that it is made out to be by the Bengaluru FSL, the accused will involuntarily answer questions posed to him during the interview.

The second fallacy is that it is incorrect to say that the accused is merely taken to the lab against his will. He is then injected with substances. The breaking of one's silence, at the time it is broken, is always technically 'voluntary'. Similarly, it can be argued that after being subject to electric shocks, a subject 'quite voluntarily' divulges information. But the act or threat of violence is where the element of coercion is housed. In narcoanalysis, the drug contained in the syringe is the element of compulsion. The rest is technically voluntary.

- In 2004, the Bombay High Court ruled in the multi-crore-rupee fake stamp paper case that subjecting an accused to certain tests like narcoanalysis does not violate the fundamental right against self-incrimination. Article 20(3) of the Constitution guarantees this, "No person accused of any offence shall be compelled to be a witness against himself." Statements made under narcoanalysis are not admissible in evidence. However, recoveries resulting from such drugged interviews are admissible as corroborative evidence. This is, arguably, a round about way to subverting the right to silence—acquiring the information on where to find the weapon from the subject, in his right senses, he would not turn witness against himself.
- Arguments have been made that narcoanalysis constitutes mental torture. It works by inhibiting the nervous system and thus lowering the subject's inhibitions. It is not difficult to interpret this as a physical violation of an individual's mind-space.
- The State Police Departments are responsible for generating demand for the process. The decision to conduct narcoanalysis is usually made by the Superintendent of Police or the Deputy Inspector General handling a case.
- Some officials connected to law enforcement argue that narcoanalysis can be of great use in instances where witnesses turned hostile; rape cases where issues of consent are being debated; and cases where the investigating officer is hard pressed for time or working to disrupt offences planned for the near future, including terrorist acts.

SCOPE FOR ABUSE

- Authorities are likely to abuse the power to decide which situations will warrant such exceptions, even when such extraordinary situations are explicitly laid out by law. It will be difficult to find a fool-proof way to determine which suspect is concealing information. These questions of discretion aside, when a country claims to be committed to human rights and against torture, one may ask if there can even be a situation that warrants a deviation from its commitment to such principles.
- While the expert studies and court opinions available internationally have granted that there may be some use in narcoanalysis, the overwhelming evidence is that narcoanalysis is by no means a reliable science. In the face of a near-consensus internationally, one or two Indian forensic labs claim to have new evidence and studies claiming remarkable success rates for the process. They must now prove their claim that narcoanalysis is backed by sound science.
- State governments need to work with the central authorities to enhance the investigative capabilities of their police departments. The police now hand over one of the most crucial parts of the investigation to a clinical psychologist conducting narcoanalysis. Interrogation is an art as well as a science. It takes enormous amounts of training and patience. The central government must make a clear policy stand on narcoanalysis – because what is at stake is India's commitment to individual freedoms and a clean criminal justice system.

INDEX

A

B

C

D

E

F

I

J

M

N

O

P

R

S

T

W